The Circle of Pregnancy

A complete and simple guide to pregnancy,
childbirth, and your child's first months.

Dr Darryl Ableman, M.B.B.Ch.

Note for Librarians: A cataloguing record for this book is available from Library and Archives Canada at www.collectionscanada.ca/amicus/index-e.html
ISBN 1-4120-9481-x

Printed in Canada.

Elba publishing
Offices in Canada
#56-2991 Lougheed Hwy Coquitlam B.C. V3B6J6
tel 604 945-7819   fax 604 945-2884
Order online at:
circleofpregnancy.com
Contact us at :
ableman2223@telus.net

10 9 8 7 6 5 4

Table of Contents

Preface

This book is dedicated to my family:

To my wife Shweed—for your enthusiasm and support over the years; for understanding my passion for my work; for selflessly compromising your freedom; for the many dates, functions and gatherings I have had to bail on.
I am forever indebted to you for your sacrifice.

To all my awesome children, Rylie, Spencer, Taylor, Makenzi—for your patience and understanding while I dragged you to so many of these deliveries and for waiting all those long hours while I was delivering 'the baby'.

And finally, to my parents for your wonderful support and encouragement through my years of study.

Introduction

I graduated from Witwatersrand University in South Africa in 1984. After surviving an internship at a local hospital in Johannesburg, I began a six-month residency training in Obstetrics. Subsequently I immigrated to Canada and practiced in rural Saskatchewan before moving to Vancouver, British Columbia.

I currently work as a primary care physician with a full office practice; you can often find me in the wee hours of the morning delivering a baby. To date, I have delivered over 2500 babies.

You may ask, if this guy is so busy delivering babies and seeing pregnant women and newborns ... why the book?

Well, besides my excellent linguistic skills and my hopes of making a fortune from writing My First Book, I recognize that all pregnant women seem to ask the same questions. I often feel that I sound like a broken answering machine, responding to the same questions again and again.

Most of the women I see are concerned parents-to-be who want to be as well educated as possible. I support their quest in finding out as much as they can.

There is a wealth of overwhelming information available on pregnancy, and so many books on the subject. It's my belief that even the bestsellers have too much redundant information; prospective parents can get lost without finding the pertinent and salient issues. It can be both overwhelming and confusing.

So I have mustered up my energy to write this book so that

11

it ALL makes sense. Here are the issues that I believe are key. Here's the meat, without all the gravy. I hope that by trimming away the excess information that is often so confusing, I can help you through your pregnancy, and eliminate any misunderstandings and fears you may have as you progress on your journey towards the birth of your child.

I would also like to explain my choice of book title. I believe that once you have fallen pregnant it changes your life forever. It has an effect that leads from one chapter of your life into an exciting new one. The circle of pregnancy is also indicative of the circle of intimacy that is created both within your family circle in addition to your circle of close friends, due to this pregnancy. The circle that is created forms a new beginning for you, your partner and your immediate family. The concept of a circle also brings a concept of stages, from the time that the thought of falling pregnant occurs to conception and then to the stages of pregnancy. From here we move into the next stages which include labour, delivery, the newborn, and perhaps the idea of further pregnancies.

Before It All Begins

You have decided to fall pregnant and want to be as proactive as possible. You want this to be an exciting adventure, and you hope you can get it right, right from the beginning.

First, you need to look at the full picture. Do not fantasize about this. The next time you are in the supermarket, take a good look at the mother and child in the checkout line. Can you see yourself in three years time, dealing with that small boy having a tantrum over the candy he wanted but didn't get? If you are still committed, read on.

Don't get me wrong. You're looking at this book on pregnancy and babies, so I assume that you do want to have children, but as a parent of four children myself, I recognize how big an investment you'll have to make. The investment covers not just the emotional and physical parts of parenthood, but sacrifices and finances as well.

So now that we've clarified that you have purchased the correct book, let's start off with what you need to do before it all begins.

If you have any medical problems, you need to sit down with your doctor ahead of time. There may be certain things that should be addressed, such as a medication that is contraindicated in pregnancy or a medical disease that requires a closer watch during the pregnancy.

Fifty years ago, when you fell pregnant you saw your doctor for visits and continued your inactive lifestyle, which likely included smoking and unrestricted amounts of alcohol intake. Just watch an old movie and note the pregnant wife with the martini in one hand and the cigarette hanging from the mouth.

Nowadays, we know about so many things that are potentially harmful that it makes sense to see a physician before it all begins so that you can be proactive.

Health and Nutrition

Let's look at your diet and exercise regime. What should you do now to establish good habits for when you are pregnant? The most important thing is to eat well so that your body can start to meet the needs of the baby once you have conceived.

This means following Canada's Food Guide, which recommends 1200 mg of calcium daily, from 3 to 4 servings of milk products. One serving of milk product could be 1 cup of milk, or 3/4 cup of yogurt, or 2 ounces of natural or processed cheese. With this much milk product intake, you'll get all your recommended vitamin D.

Remember that different people need different amounts of food, depending on age, body size, activity level, male or female, pregnant or breastfeeding. That's why the Food Guide gives a lower and higher number of servings for each food group. For example, young children can choose the lower number of servings, while male teenagers can go to the higher number. Most other people can choose servings somewhere in between. Pregnant women require additional iron, protein, zinc, folic acid and vitamin B, so be sure to eat red meat, chicken, fish, dry beans, eggs, and nuts on a regular basis.

The tables below should give you some ideas for your new and improved diet:

Grain Products	Vegetables and Fruit	Milk Products	Meat and Alternatives
Choose whole grain and enriched products more often.	Choose dark green and orange vegetables and orange fruit more often.	Choose lower-fat milk products more often.	Choose leaner meats, poultry and fish, as well as dried peas, beans, and lentils more often.

Grain Products 5-12 SERVINGS PER DAY

1 Serving: Cold Cereal 1 Slice, 30 g; Hot Cereal 175 mL 3/4 cup

2 Servings: 1 Bagel, Pita or Bun; Pasta or Rice 250 mL 1 cup

Vegetables & Fruit 5-10 SERVINGS PER DAY

1 Serving: 1 Medium Size Vegetable or Fruit; Fresh, Frozen or Canned Vegetables or Fruit 125 mL 1/2 cup; Salad 250 mL 1 cup; Juice 125 mL 1/2 cup

Milk Products SERVINGS PER DAY
Children 4–9 years: 2–3
Youth 10–16 years: 3–4
Adults: 2–4
Pregnant & Breast-feeding Women: 3–4

1 Serving: Milk 250 mL 1 cup; Cheese 3"x1"x1" 50 g, 2 Slices 50 g; Yogourt 175 g 3/4 cup

Other Foods

Taste and enjoyment can also come from other foods and beverages that are not part of the 4 food groups. Some of these foods are higher in fat or Calories, so use these foods in moderation.

Meat & Alternatives 2-3 SERVINGS PER DAY

1 Serving: Meat, Poultry or Fish 50–100 g; Fish 1/3–2/3 Can 50–100 g; 1-2 Eggs; Beans 125-250 mL; Tofu 100 g 1/3 cup; Peanut Butter 30 mL 2 tbsp

So what does this really mean in the real world? Sometimes when I look at the tables, I get really confused. Does this mean that you should start eating for two?

As a general rule, the logical approach is to keep a healthy, well-balanced, 1800-calorie diet. This means eating 3 well-balanced meals, each containing 4 grams of meat, a portion of pasta, rice, potato or bread for carbohydrates, and finally vegetables.

Your exercise routine does not need to be complicated, but you should get 30 minutes of aerobic exercise 3 days a week. As your pregnancy advances, you can adapt and modify this program. I will go into more detail on exercise in pregnancy once you are there.

Finally consider these key points before falling pregnant:

♦ Prenatal vitamins (Materna or PregVit) can be started at this point.
♦ Make sure that you have quit smoking. If you need help with this, see your family doctor.
♦ Ideally, you should not drink alcohol once you have conceived, so why not quit drinking alcohol now.
♦ If you own a cat, have someone else change the litter from now on. Cat litter is home to a parasite that can cause toxoplasmosis in your fetus in its early stages.
♦ If you have a history of hepatitis B or C, syphilis, or HIV/ AIDS, notify your doctor of your plans to fall pregnant. Check to make sure that you are immune to chickenpox, rubella and measles. If you are unsure, there are blood tests that can help.
♦ Avoid ingestion of unpasteurized milk and milk products, and of honey.
♦ If you were on the pill, allow yourself a normal period, and then you may attempt to fall pregnant. Should you become pregnant while you are still on the pill, stop taking it as soon as possible. This is not unusual and is certainly no cause for concern.
♦ If you use an Intra Uterine Device (IUD), this must be removed before you try to conceive.

♦ If your workplace exposes you to any toxins or your work is physically very strenuous, talk to your doctor so that some form of plan can be worked out ahead of time.

NEWLY PREGNANT...
So You're Pregnant ... Now What?

Yahoo! The home pregnancy test turns out to be positive! You are finally pregnant, and now after waiting patiently you are seeing the doctor who delivers babies. You can hardly wait to hear all the things that you will need. But instead, you are sitting in front of a doctor who congratulates you ... and then tells you to come back when you are 12 weeks pregnant for your first prenatal exam. You are shocked! There must be more to this visit! Perhaps your doctor doesn't understand what's going on!

The reality is that even though so much is happening in the development of the fetus at the embryonic and cellular level in the first 12 weeks of your pregnancy, there just is not too much to it on your end. I am not trying to sound negative about your new exciting gift. The truth is that nobody wishes to hear the bad stuff. So, please don't be offended by my next statement. One in five women will unfortunately have a natural miscarriage in the first 12 weeks—not because of any bad things she did before finding out she was pregnant, but because of the laws of nature. That's the reason we try to avoid doing the first prenatal exam until we are somewhat guaranteed that this vulnerable stage is likely to be over. Thus, the first official pregnancy visit is the 12th-week first prenatal visit. That said, I generally try to establish a few things during your initial visit to me.

First, let's see if you are truly pregnant. A positive reading is usually determined eight days after conception. Urine tests vary in the way they test positive for pregnancy. Some have a 'control' that shows you what the test part should look like if it is positive. Others change colour or have a negative or blank space that will develop into a +/plus sign if you are pregnant.

If urine is too diluted, pregnancy is sometimes not detected. The urine of a pregnant woman contains the hormone human chorionic gonadotropin (HCG), which is produced by the growing placenta and fetus. The hormone is easier to detect if the urine is concentrated, which is why the first morning urine is the most effective. I am often faced with a urine pregnancy test with a very faint positive line that is not easily detected. I have even found myself in a situation where the woman has tested positive three times at home and wanted official confirmation. When we tested her, the test was negative because we saw her when the HCG in her urine was more diluted.

If your periods are usually very regular, but you've missed one, there could be many reasons other than pregnancy for missing it. If I am uncertain why you are not testing positive, I can order a quantitative b-HCG blood test, which is very accurate in detecting pregnancy. If this is not an available option, another urine test can be done one week later.

The next thing we need to do is to figure out how many weeks pregnant you are.

This is calculated not from the day you conceived but from the first day of your last menstrual period (LMP). In reality, a pregnancy will usually last 38 weeks. Because we are adding two weeks at the beginning, the pregnancy lasts around 40 weeks. We then allow a further ten days over the due date.

Most women will go over their expected date of delivery

(EDD) so as a mind-set I advise patients to avoid disappointment early by calculating the worst-case scenario and then adding ten days to their due date. This way, the longest period they are going to be pregnant is established.

What else?

Diet

Diet in pregnancy is very simple. Keep in mind that you are the *host* to this growing baby, and it will generally take whatever it needs from you at your expense. Because of this, healthy babies are born in all nations of the world, regardless of how good a diet the mother's socio-economic status allows her.

There are, however, some crucial additional little things. This should include taking 1 mg of folic acid daily in the first 12 weeks, as this has been shown to reduce the chance of neural tube defects and spina bifida, in which a portion of the spinal cord does not close.

It is also important to take 1200 mg of calcium and 5 mcg (micrograms) of vitamin D in your daily diet to avoid osteoporosis in later life. Lastly you should be on a diet high enough in iron to avoid anemia in pregnancy. Make sure you get 30 mg every day.

Many women take a general pregnancy vitamin to supplement them throughout the pregnancy. In spite of this, I find that many women end up needing additional iron in the last twelve weeks in the amount of 300 to 900 mg of ferrous gluconate daily for anemia. One of the practical difficulties in making a perfect pregnancy vitamin is allowing enough iron, but not too much, otherwise constipation becomes a problem.

In pregnancy, healthy eating is important to your overall general feeling of wellbeing. It is often initially difficult, however, to keep up with three full meals a day, especially with nausea in its different forms of severity. It therefore often makes sense to eat as many small meals a day as you need to feel comfortable.

Probably the most important issue to address is weight gain, which I will discuss in itself later on. In terms of your diet, however, the usual scenario I see is the 28-week-pregnant mother who greets me in tears because she is fat! She doesn't eat anything and yet she is already 40 pounds heavier. Then she adds, that in addition to her scant diet, she likes to drink two litres of *no-sugar-added, all-natural fruit juice*—which contains 2000 calories of fructose. Those 2000 calories are notoriously the culprit. So my rule of *no juice or pop* is implemented at the first visit. Instead, drink 6 to 8 glasses of water daily.

Avoid unpasteurized milk and milk products, because they can contain bacteria that can cause a miscarriage. The chance that you will be drinking unpasteurized milk products is slim to none, unless you live in rural areas.

Research has shown that some seafoods, especially swordfish, mackerel, shark and tuna, contain high traces of mercury. This can potentially harm a fetus, so cut down on seafood. You do not have to stop eating it completely, as you would have to ingest reasonably large quantities in order for the mercury to pose a problem. The FDA recommends eating no more than one tin of tuna per week. Raw fish, shellfish and sushi may all contain parasites that potentially infect the mother and take certain nutrients from her, but which do not directly harm the baby.

Again, undercooked meats and poultry can cause parasitic infection that may do the same as the raw fish, but I am more concerned with infection with bacteria that may have more serious effects on the baby.

High amounts of nitrites are found in sausage, bacon and deli meats; try to avoid these, or eat them only in moderation

Morning Sickness (hyperemesis gravidarum)

In considering food, we also need to consider that for many newly pregnant women this is the furthest thing from their minds, and for them, morning sickness should be called 'all-day-and-night sickness'. It is seen as early as the fifth week and is caused by rising levels of b-HCG, the hormone produced by the fetus and placenta. There are different degrees of nausea; some may require simple measures such as limiting your choices of foods, while others may need to be controlled with specific oral anti-nausea drugs such as Diclectin®. Some women may even require hospitalization for intravenous rehydration and antinauseants. Morning sickness usually disappears between the 12th and 14th weeks, although it can go on for longer. On occasion, I have seen women who have had to continue with their medication throughout the pregnancy.

If Diclectin has failed, Gravol® and Stemetil® may be used. Although they are not exclusively for pregnancy-induced nausea, neither are harmful to the baby.

Weight Gain

How much weight gain can you allow in pregnancy? How does each part of the baby contribute? Most women on average will gain about 30-40 pounds over the course of their pregnancy. A general rule may be applied: if you are underweight, you should try to gain more; if you are overweight, you should try to gain less. There are obvious exceptions such as twin or multiple pregnancies where woman will gain more. However, it becomes confusing for both mother and doctor when you try to adhere to a week-by-week weight-gain schedule because babies cannot read. As a rule patients do not always follow an expected weight gain pattern, and this can cause a great deal of worry. My practical approach is, try to eat as much of a well-balanced, healthy meal as possible.

Avoid fast foods. Don't worry if you gain a lot of weight one month. But if you do, then you need to go back and look at the reason. If you can't explain the increase, perhaps there is a medical reason. Perhaps your diet is high in salt, leading to fluid retention, or you may have a big baby due to gestational diabetes, or you may have twins, or you may have too much amniotic fluid (poly-hydramnios).

All that said and done, you are still going to ask how much weight is the norm. So at the onset, you would calculate your Body Mass Index (BMI), which is your height in centimeters (inches) divided by your mass weight in kilograms (pounds) respectively.

If you have a BMI of <20, you are underweight; 13 to 18 kg total weight gain with weekly 2nd and 3rd trimester weight gain of 1/2 kg per week is recommended. Similarly, with a BMI of 20-25, you are a normal weight; 11 to 16 kg total weight gain with 2nd and 3rd trimester weekly weight gain of 0.3-0.4 kg is recommended. A BMI of 25-27 means you are overweight; you require a total weight gain of 7 to 11 kg with 2nd and 3rd trimester weekly weight gain of 1/4 kg. A BMI of >27 means you are obese. A total weight gain of 7 to 9 kg is needed, *and* a consultation with a dietitian.

So what makes you gain weight? There are many contributors:

Baby	3.5 kg/7.5 lb
Amniotic fluid	1.0 kg/2 lb
Blood	2 kg/4 lb
Breast	1.5 kg/3 lb
Placenta	0.5 kg/1 lb
Uterus	1 kg/2.5 lb

Finally, the body needs extra stores for breastfeeding and pregnancy of 2.5 to 3.5 kg/5 to 8 lb.

Any weight above and beyond this is fat.

Maternity Vitamins and Minerals

Maternity vitamins should be taken as directed—never take extra amounts of prenatal vitamins, as the recommended daily allowance of vitamin A is present in each tablet, and levels of more than 10 000 IU of vitamin A are toxic and dangerous to the developing baby. In fact, high doses of vitamin A are linked to birth defects. For this very reason, do not eat liver while you are pregnant. The recommended daily allowance of calcium is 1200 mg and 200 IU, or 5 mcg, of vitamin D. Maternity vitamins usually contain about 250 mg and 250 IU respectively.

Alcohol and Smoking

How about alcohol and cigarettes? Well, these are two habits that you need to stop immediately. There is often much concern about these prior to finding out about the pregnancy. It's preferable to stop when you are planning to conceive, but if you did not, *don't sweat it! Just stop now.* There is a direct correlation between cigarette smoking and low birth weight and premature babies. Further, infants and children are harmed by secondhand smoke. This is why you should quit smoking if you are pregnant and an established smoker. It is a prerequisite for a healthy future for your child.

A further incentive is that if you can quit before your 16th week, there is less chance of a small baby or preterm labour. There can often be a weird rationalization that if the baby is smaller, it is better for the delivery. The problem is that after the baby is born, he or she is going to be more prone to illness, and sleeping and eating problems.

Alcohol is directly linked to a disorder called fetal alcohol syndrome (FAS). Babies with FAS are characterized by being smaller than normal, and tend to have facial, eye, and ear abnormalities. They may also have heart defects, poor coordination and developmental delays or learning problems. Behavioral problems are often seen, such as hyperactivity, impulsive behavior, and a poor attention span. These effects are permanent. They are also avoidable by abstaining from alcohol while pregnant. The difficulty is in knowing how much alcohol it takes to do this. There is *no* known safe level of alcohol use in pregnancy and therefore to be safe, you should stop drinking alcohol entirely once you find out you are pregnant. Ideally, you should stop as soon as you are preparing to fall pregnant.

Exercise

Exercise is important in pregnancy as long as you don't have another medical condition such as high blood pressure or a heart condition, etc. I tell my patients to listen to their bodies. Don't start doing something radically different just because you are pregnant and don't stop doing an activity unless it hurts or it becomes difficult.

Stop contact sports after the baby is no longer confined to the pelvis (i.e., after 12 weeks). The rationale is that the fetus can be traumatized once the uterus has expanded outside of the boney protective pelvis and into the abdominal cavity.

I always think of one particular patient as an example of exercise during pregnancy. She taught aerobics in the days of high impact and bounced through all three pregnancies until going into labour while teaching on all three occasions.

Some general rules that I have touched on may be universally applied. So keep active as tolerated but don't suddenly try to do something radical that is going to stress your body.

If you are a competitive athlete, then you will need to maybe slow down as the pregnancy progresses. For those who have not been active, you can begin a walking program and increase your distance and pace as you tolerate it. Remember that you should keep well hydrated because you produce more heat during pregnancy. Limit your activity during hot humid weather.

Exercise mild to moderately three times a week for thirty minutes as tolerated. If you weight train, then modify this by reducing your weights and increasing the number of repetitions. Avoid lying on your back without something like a wedge beneath you to create an angle to avoid compromising blood flow to the baby. This becomes more crucial as the pregnancy progresses.

Learn to recognize signs that indicate that you need to stop or slow down. These include dizziness, rapid heart beat, swollen ankles, swollen feet, swollen calves, headaches, nausea, vomiting or vaginal bleeding.

Learn the correct procedure for lying down or getting up. To lie down, first bend your knees. Then kneel down on one knee while placing your hand on the other thigh for extra support. Then bring the other knee down so that you are kneeling on both knees, and at the same time lean forward so that your arms and hands are partially supporting you. Now take your weight on your arms to help you slide onto your side. Then ease your way onto your back using the strength of your arms. When getting up, reverse the steps that you used to lie down.

Stretching exercises

These will reduce muscle tension, but they will also improve flexibility. Each person has a starting point of flexibility, so if you feel pain during a stretch, stop it or do it less rigorously.

The general rule for stretching is to breathe with each stretch. This helps you relax. Hold each position for 20 to 60 seconds. Always follow a stretch on one side by the same on the other side. And remember, if it hurts, you are doing it wrong.

Shoulders and back stretch

Face the wall with your knees slightly bent and your feet apart and in line with your hips. Place your hands against the wall above your head. Then tilt your pelvis inward towards the wall.

Shoulders and chest stretch

Stand sideways, close to a wall. Bring your arm up to the wall at shoulder height with your palm against the wall, but not pushing against it. Repeat with the other arm.

Calf stretch

With your hips square and your feet facing the wall, extend one leg behind you. Balance your body leaning with your forearms against the wall. Repeat with the other leg.

Quadriceps stretch

Leaning against the wall with your palm, bend your opposite knee and grab hold of your foot with your hand on the same side. Repeat on the other side.

Hamstring stretch

Sit on a desk, couch or bench and stretch one leg out to a fully extended position. Keep your back straight and bend forward slightly from your lower spine. There should be a tightening or burning of the muscle in the back of the upper leg. It is not necessary to reach to your feet. Repeat on the other side.

Back stretch

This relieves back pain in pregnancy. Kneel on your hands and knees, with your elbows slightly bent. Keep your back flat. Then round your back up at the same time that you tighten your abdominal and buttock muscles. Slowly relax and allow your back to return to the flat position. This can be repeated up to 10 to 15 times.

Strengthening exercises

In order to prepare for childbirth, you need to strengthen your muscles. There are various types of exercises to help with this.

Kegel exercises

Kegel exercises strengthen the vaginal and perineal areas for birth and after birth. They can be done standing or sitting, until you are more than 4 months pregnant, when you should do them standing.

Tighten the muscles around the vagina and anus, as you would if you were waiting to urgently use the bathroom. Hold this contraction for as long as is comfortable. Increase the time that you do this to 8 to 10 seconds and try to reach a goal of doing this about 25 times a day.

Squatting is a position often used in labour. It uses many muscles groups, so you need to strengthen them all to make it easier on these groups when they are really needed.

Position your back against the wall for support. The feet should be comfortably placed away from the wall and more than hip-width apart. Keep them flat on the floor. As you squat, use the wall for back support and allow your buttocks to move down to the floor. If you have knee trouble, do not try a deep squat as this will cause your kneecap to really hurt. You should try to hold a squat for 30 to 60 seconds.

Wall pushups

Stand facing the wall and place your hands out in front of you against the wall at shoulder height, and shoulder-width apart. Keep your back straight, your pelvis tilted down, and your knees slightly bent. Now bend at your elbows and bring yourself closer to the wall. Breathe in at the same time. Then extend your elbows and push your body away from the wall. Breathe out while doing this. This will strengthen the triceps and pectoralis muscles.

Thigh stretching and strengthening exercises

Stretching the inner thigh muscles will help you during labour. Sit with your legs apart with your back against a wall for extra support if needed. Your knees should be out and your feet touching at the soles. Place your hands under the knees and gently press both knees towards the floor without using your hands. Hold this for 10 to 20 seconds.

Then repeat, but this time, use your hands to resist the downward motion of your knees. Do this for 10 to 20 seconds.

Abdominal exercises for stomach-muscle strengthening

Stomach-muscle separation is also known as rectus muscle diastasis. This may occur in any pregnant woman as the uterus expands, resulting in pressure behind the abdominal muscles. If the tissue between the two bands of rectus muscle weakens too much, a softness occurs between these two bands in the midline. If you lie on your back with your knees bent and lift your head off the floor by 15 to 20 cm, you can see this. It is not a big deal and is common. It will not affect your ability to do your strengthening exercises.

Stomach muscle tightening

Lie on your back with knees bent. Breathe out while pulling in your abdominal muscles and pressing the curve of your lower back into the floor. Then relax and breathe in. This may be increased to

8 to 10 repetitions.

Modified crunches

If you are in your first trimester, lie flat on your back. If you are in your second or third trimester, keep a 45-degree incline. Keep your knees bent. Breathe in and place your hands on your abdomen. Lift your shoulders slightly off the ground, and breathe out while pushing your lower back into the floor. Hold this position for two normal breaths and then slowly lower your head to the floor and relax. Start with six repetitions and increase with time as tolerated.

Drugs and Medications

There is a great deal of confusion about which medications are safe to take in pregnancy. In my opinion it often comes down to medical liability. There isn't a single drug company that will stipulate that the drug that you are about to take is safe in pregnancy. In this way, the companies avoid legal blame down the road. Diclectin which is a Canadian produced morning sickness anti-nausea medication is essentially the only drug that is specifically formulated for pregnancy.

The following list shows the very few medications that are absolutely prohibited in pregnancy: the oral anti-acne drug Accutane®, tetracyclic antibiotics, anticonvulsants (such as Phenytoin and Valproic acid), Quinine (for leg cramps), Coumadin® (a blood thinner), and lithium (for manic depression), and several other categories such as antihypertensive treatments (ACE inhibitors).

Most selective serotonin reuptake inhibitor (SSRI) antidepressant medications have been thought to be safe in pregnancy. Most recently, however, a study of 3,581 pregnant women has shown that in first-trimester patients there is an increased risk of overall congenital malformations as well as cardiovascular malformations especially if the patient was taking Paxil® or paroxetine. This raises the issue that if a previously depressed patient wishes to fall pregnant, she needs to consider discontinuation of her SSRI in the first trimester. The pros and cons obviously need to be considered.

I will always remember the patient who came to me to refer her for terminating her third pregnancy after I had delivered her previous two babies. She thought she should do this because before she knew she was pregnant, she had consumed alcohol and taken an anti-depressant and had visions of an abnormal baby as a result. Her third baby turned out just fine. With the correct information, her fears were allayed.

Prescribed drugs that fit into a grey area are too many to mention. These medications are not teratogenic. This means that they do not produce deformities, so they have never been proven bad, but there are no studies to show they are officially safe. For this reason, the pros and cons and the trade offs need to be taken into consideration by both doctor and patient.

Most over-the-counter (OTC) medications are totally safe, although Ibuprofen (Advil®, Motrin®) is not advised in the first and last trimester. Tylenol® and codeine are safe. Anti-ulcer medication like Zantac®, and antihistamines that are free of pseudoepinephrine and epinephrine are safe, for example, Benadryl®, Chlor-Tripolon®, Claritin®, Reactine®. Most cough medications have dextromorphan, which is a codeine derivative that is safe, as long it is not combined with pseudoepinephrine and epinephrine. Aspirin® (ASA) is not harmful and is often used in women with recurrent miscarriages and with the autoimmune disease lupus. It should be stopped at 36 weeks to avoid an increased chance of bleeding during and after labour, because aspirin inhibits the stickiness of platelets. If stopped at 36 weeks the platelets will function normally within two weeks and therefore the chance of heavy vaginal bleeding is minimized.

Herbs should not be taken unless they are discussed first with your doctor. Black cohosh specifically is harmful during pregnancy and should be avoided.

The last group of drugs to discuss is street drugs. These include marijuana, cocaine (crack), amphetamines, methamphetamines (crystal meths), LSD (lysergic acid), and benzodiazepines. These are all harmful to a developing fetus and are contraindicated.

The effects of each drug vary, but cocaine and its derivatives are especially fatal in that they constrict the blood vessels to the placenta and may result in a separation of the placenta called abruptio placenta.

Caffeine

It is safe to drink coffee up to three cups a day. One study has shown an increase chance of miscarriage in women who consumed more than three cups a day. Tea contains caffeine as well as tannins and so should be treated as for coffee. Be aware of certain herbal teas such as green tea, ginseng and similar teas, which are harmful during pregnancy. Safe herbal teas are berry varieties, citrus-flavored teas and peppermint and chamomile teas.

Investigations

Tests such as an ultrasound have very little benefit in the early stages other than to establish a cause of bleeding, or the dates of the baby (when the dates are impossible for the woman to establish herself), or in suspected twin or multiple pregnancies, or when trying to exclude an ectopic pregnancy, which is a pregnancy that occurs outside of the uterus and in the fallopian tube.

Your Pregnancy and The Facts

Choosing a Caregiver

Who should be involved in delivering your baby? This will vary from one country to another and sometimes from one city to the next. In British Columbia, Canada, there are many available options.

In an ideal model, the family physician should be the primary caregiver for the pregnant woman, provide prenatal care, and deliver the baby, as well as being involved in the post-delivery care of both the mom and the baby. This used to be the most common case. However, family practice has changed so much over the years, and fewer and fewer family physicians choose to be involved in primary care obstetrics. Now we have primary care obstetric clinics with several family physicians who work within the clinic and deliver patients according to a designated call schedule within the hospital obstetric unit.

The unfortunate part of this set-up is that continuity of care has been lost. In other communities, such as Ontario, there are obstetricians/gynecologists who do primary care obstetrics and who are involved in delivery of obstetrical care, but again this is their only function.

At the end of the day, the woman is somewhat lost in that she doesn't have a primary care physician who continues to provide her with care for herself and her newborn baby.

In many other countries, midwives perform the duties of a primary caregiver for both prenatal and postnatal care. The drawback of this system is that midwives need to refer the patient to a physician for anything that is medical, which can often lead to a doubling up of services as the doctor is not really involved in the care of the mom. There is also the issue once again of who is to care for the newborn.

In Canada, in addition to midwives, mothers can choose the services of a doula. Unlike a doctor or midwife, doulas are not qualified to deliver babies. They can, however, provide a very good emotional support system, especially where such a system is absent, but it is sometimes difficult to judge in advance whether their services are going to be beneficial or not.

Some maternity units provide an early-labour-at-home service using nurses with midwife training. This support service can be extremely useful to the mother before the need to come in to the hospital becomes pressing.

All in all, it becomes somewhat confusing for a pregnant woman when she is trying to make the best choice in care for herself and her baby.

I believe that the most important thing is to find someone who will be involved in the care of the pregnant mother throughout her pregnancy, will continue to follow her after the baby is born, and will be involved with the baby. If you have a physician or midwife who can provide this form of care, stick with that person as they are truly a rarity.

The next most crucial aspect is to find someone you can communicate with, who makes you feel both comfortable and confident.

To Tell or Not

Perhaps you have the notion that you should keep you pregnancy to yourself and your partner until you are further along. This way, if something goes wrong you will deal with it in private. I disagree. I don't see the point of thinking this way. By keeping your pregnancy to yourself, you're keeping a secret. Pregnancy is not something to be embarrassed about, it is a very exciting time, and by sharing the news with your friends and family, you are inviting the people who are central to your life to experience your joy and happiness. In the same way they can also share in any disappointment and upset that can arise if anything unfortunate happens. Grieving a miscarriage alone is very difficult and it is even more difficult to share things after the fact. If your friends and family have shared in your joy and excitement, it will be far easier for them to share in your loss and be supportive for you.

Your First Prenatal Visit

So, now that you have found someone who will follow you through your pregnancy, deliver your baby, and optimally look after you and your newborn, you should see him or her at the 12-week mark for your first prenatal visit.

At this visit, you will be examined to see how your baby is growing and whether there are any risk issues that need to be addressed immediately. Your doctor or midwife will do a first assessment based on your medical and family history, followed by a physical examination. You will need to provide details of your family history for inherited diseases such as Tay-Sachs disease, or thalassemia or other ethnic diseases.

You also need to talk about whether you have any risk factors such as diabetes or hypertension, or any medical diseases such as hepatitis or HIV/AIDS that may affect the baby.

The assessment also includes listening to the fetal heart for the first time. This is usually an extremely happy time for all because it seems to validate and confirm all the changes that have occurred up to now.

If the due date of the baby is known, based on the first day of the last menstrual period, an ultrasound is not necessary, unless there are other concerns such as twin pregnancy or fetal viability or implantation concerns. Ultrasound otherwise only becomes necessary to establish the growth and development of a baby between 18 to 20 weeks. Sex is easier to identify at 20 weeks.

I generally do not do blood work at 12 weeks because at this point it will only confirm the presence of risk factors that we do not need to be aware of until the time of birth. I wait another four weeks so that the mother need only have one set of blood tests done all at the same time. The only exception to this is if the woman is less than 16 weeks pregnant and has had bleeding vaginally. It then becomes necessary to see she is Rh-negative and if so to give a Rhogam® shot. This is usually done in a hospital setting where Rh tests and Rhogam are readily available.

Triple Screen Test

As I said, I generally do all the blood tests at one go, at 16 weeks. The blood tests include a panel for thyroid disease (TSH), anemia (CBC), immunity to rubella and chickenpox, exposure to sexually transmitted diseases (STDs), such as syphilis (VDRL test), HIV/AIDS, hepatitis B and C, and Triple Screen Test. Triple screen can give us information similar to that we would get from doing an amniocentesis at 15 to 16 weeks. Because this is a blood test, however, it spares the patient the risk of the complications of amniocentesis such as cramping or fetal demise. The drawback is that it can test false positive, and we will discuss this later. The test measures the levels of three proteins that are made by the baby or the placenta, and are found in the mother's blood. These three proteins are:

♦ **AFP:** alpha-fetoprotein
♦ **uE3:** uncongugated estriol
♦ **hCG:** human chorionic gonadotropin

The levels of these proteins are different in some pregnancies affected with Down syndrome, Open Spina Bifida, or Trisomy 18. The differences in these protein levels are used to estimate the risk to each individual pregnancy.

In general, the triple screen test can create quite a bit of anxiety as it is available from 15+ weeks of pregnancy, and it is usually done to test whether the mother has a baby with a Neural tube defect (N.T.D), Trisomy 18 or Down syndrome.

Neural defects can come in various forms such as anencephaly or spina bifida and is often called Spina Bifida. This defect occurs when the spine does not completely close around the spinal cord. This opening in the spine, leaves the spinal cord exposed, which results in nerve damage of varying degree. People with Open Spina Bifida can have paralysis or problems walking, and may have learning disabilities and bowel and bladder control difficulties. Anencephaly is a more severe NTD, in which the brain and skull do not develop properly. Babies with anencephaly cannot survive outside the womb.

Down syndrome is also called trisomy 21 in which there is a third copy of the 21st chromosome. This extra chromosome is the cause of their condition. Individuals with Down syndrome have:

♦ Mild to moderate mental disability
♦ specific facial features
♦ may have heart abnormalities

♦ may have other physical disabilities

Trisomy 18 is a chromosome abnormality in which an individual has an extra copy of the 18th chromosome. Individuals with trisomy 18 have severe mental and physical disabilities. The majority of babies with trisomy 18 do not survive past a few days or weeks of life. There is unfortunately no cure for this condition.

In the past, the tests for Down syndrome, Trisomy 18 and Neural tube defects were only done in women over 35. Recently, the tests have become available for all pregnancies to screen for these anomalies so that the parents can then determine whether they wish to terminate the pregnancy or not.

If the parents are committed to going through with their pregnancy regardless of what the nature of their baby is going to be, my general advice is to avoid amniocentesis or triple screen testing as you wouldn't do anything about any potential abnormality that the test might reveal.

I have several patients who have had Down syndrome babies and they are darling and loving patients, but there are many families who do not wish to have a challenged child and have chosen to terminate the pregnancy under the circumstances. This is their choice, and as a physician, I do not judge them for their choices. They are the ones who are faced with the challenge of living with this decision, and I support them in whichever way I can by providing them with the options available.

The first thing I do is to establish whether the parents would do anything to alter the pregnancy if the fetus is abnormal. If the parents wouldn't do anything, but would want to be emotionally and psychologically prepared, then I believe it is worth doing a triple screen test.

All patients under the age of 35 get a triple screen test at 15 weeks of their pregnancy. In British Columbia we have a result within two weeks. A positive screening test gives laws of probability that there is a one-in-so-many chance of their baby being a Down-syndrome or spina-bifida baby, but it doesn't *confirm* that that is the case. In addition, false positive tests are more likely when dates are inaccurate by 8 days or more. Thus, if a screening test is positive, the patient is then compelled to do an amniocentesis. The screening test also gives a quantitative measure of positivity—in other words, it tells us whether the chances of the baby having Down syndrome are 1 in 30, or 1 in 300. This obviously will also have a predictive value on whether the patient should or shouldn't have an amniocentesis. The beauty of a triple screen test is that if it is negative, then it is negative. There is no such thing as a false negative test as long as the dates are correct. Therefore, if it's negative, it tells us that the mother is not having a baby who has any chance of having Down syndrome, Trisomy 18 or a Neural tube defect.

There is an increased probability of false positive triple screen tests for a pregnant woman 35 years and older. Because this will compel an amniocentesis, I generally recommend an amniocentesis for all those women who are going to be 35 years old by the time they deliver.

Because of advances in expertise and ultrasound technology, the chance that amniocentesis can cause a miscarriage or fatal demise is now remote, although not unknown. The chance of miscarriage with amniocentesis is 1-2 in 200 patients (i.e.0.5-1 %).

With the newer tests mentioned below there is a predicted change about to occur in many centers. The newer additional tests will result in a 50% reduction in false positive tests for Down syndrome and this in turn will reduce the need to turn to amniocentesis and other invasive means to predict Down syndrome.

There are many other tests that are either in their infancy or shortly to become available. For example, chorionic villus sampling (CVS) obtains and analyzes the baby's chromosomes and can detect abnormalities early on, but requires a needle biopsy through the cervix. This is obtained by passing a tube through the vagina and cervix to the outside of the amniotic sac to obtain a sample of the chorionic villus, which is part of the developing baby. This kind of test is quite advanced and often not available in many centres.

The main advantage of CVS, which is routinely performed at 10 or 11 weeks, is that it provides results that are often available sooner than those from amniocentesis, which is usually done between 16 and 18 weeks. The main disadvantage is that there is a higher risk to the baby in miscarrying. It is important to recognize that CVS, like amniocentesis, only counts chromosomes and therefore cannot give us any information about individual genetics. So for example, a mother can have tests done, show normal results, but still end up having a baby with clubfoot or another genetic disorder.

To add to an already complicated issue, there are further tests on the horizon. For example, newer tests are available that would help in further detecting Down syndrome in the form of a fourth marker blood test.This test is now being introduced in British Columbia but is available in many centers in North America. The 4th marker is also a protein called pregnancy associated plasma protein-A or PAPP-A. This can be performed between 10-13 weeks and will reduce the false positive rate especially in women over age 35. It currently is not available to everyone in B.C. but is being made available to high risk groups such as women of 38 yrs or more at time of delivery, previous child with trisomy 21(Down syndrome), and women 35 yrs or more at delivery with a history of recurrent miscarriage.

There is another non-interventional means of assessing Down-syndrome risk in the form of an ultrasound to assess fetal detail and measure the neck folds to determine nuchal thickness and translucency. It is also called a NT test (Nuchal Translucency). This form of ultrasound is quite intricate and would require extra training by the ultrasonographer. It is also now being used in B.C. at 11-14 weeks gestation. It is indicated in the high risk groups and women age 40 and over. It is further used in all forms of multiple pregnancy (i.e. more than one fetus)

Which tests to have? In general, I don't believe that the newer tests are necessary for parents who are low risk and already have all the current tests available to them. However if you are in the higher risk groups or have tested positive the non- invasive new tests are very promising for reducing false positive tests and providing us with detail that is reassuring to both the mother and the doctor.

Frequency of visits

How often should you see your doctor during your pregnancy? Assuming this is a normal pregnancy, after the first prenatal visit in week 12, I will see my patients once a month until the 28th week. Frequency then increases to every 2 weeks until the last month when visits become weekly.

What happens in these visits and why? We assess the growth and development of the baby and ascertain if there are any concerns for the baby and any medical complications in the expectant mother.

Each visit involves a urine sample. We are looking for the presence in the urine of sugar or protein. This could indicate the beginning of diabetes in pregnancy (gestational diabetes) or the start of a condition called pre-eclampsia (toxemia of pregnancy). We weigh you, in order to have an ongoing record of your weight to establish how the pregnancy is going. We take your blood pressure, to assess the presence of another condition called hypertension in pregnancy. Finally we listen to the baby's heartbeat and measure the uterus to establish how well the pregnancy is advancing.

Growth and Development

How big is my baby and is he fully developed? We often hear the terms embryo and fetus used interchangeably, when they are in fact different entities. An embryo is less than 9 weeks old, while a fetus is 9 weeks or more. The embryonic period (from the 4th week to the 8th week) is the most important period of human development because it marks the beginning of all major external and internal structural development.

Before this period, changes occur at the cellular level with fertilization and formation of a bilaminar embryo at 2 weeks and a trilaminar embryo in the 3rd week. These are just fancy names denoting the stages of cell development and the establishment of embryonic membranes and germ layers (ectoderm, mesoderm and endoderm).

At 4 weeks—the beginning of the embryonic period—the heart begins to beat. At the end of the 8th week—the end of the embryonic period—all the essential external and internal structures are present and have begun to evolve. At this stage, the embryo is 30 mm long.

The fetal period extends from the 9th week to the actual time of birth. During this period, rapid body growth and organ system changes take place. At the 9th week, the external genitalia show male characteristics, but the fetus may still be mistaken for female, especially using ultrasound. The sex is distinguishable at 12 weeks. Initially, head growth is rapid and then slows down in relation to the rest of the body. Lanugo (black body hair) and head hair appear, and the skin is coated with a white cheesy substance called vernix caseosa by the 20th week. The eyelids are fused during most of the fetal period but begin to open at about 26 weeks. Up to this point, the fetus has immature lungs and is thus not capable of living outside of the uterus.

Up to the 30th week, the fetus has a thin skin and a relative absence of subcutaneous fat, which results in a reddish appearance. During the last 6 to 8 weeks, fat begins to develop in the subcutaneous layer making the fetus smooth and plump. This terminal period is devoted mainly to building up tissues and preparing the systems involved in the transition from the intrauterine to the extra uterine environment.

Fetuses born prematurely during the 26th to 36th week period may survive, but full-term fetuses have the best chance of survival. The average 26-week baby will weigh about 1000 grams and will grow by about 1000 grams every four weeks to reach a weight of 3500 grams at 38 weeks. After this, the rate dramatically plateaus out. The average length of a term baby is 52 cm. By full term the percentage of white fat in the body is about 16 percent. The fetus lays down about 14 grams of fat a day during the last few weeks of pregnancy. In general, male fetuses grow faster than females and also weigh more.

Changes occurring during the fetal period are not as dramatic as those in the embryonic period but they are very important. The fetus is far less vulnerable to the teratogenic effects of drugs, viruses, and radiation, but these agents may interfere with normal functional development, especially of the brain.

Additional Tests Over the Duration of the Pregnancy

An ultrasound is routinely done at 18 to 20 weeks to determine fetal growth and development, and at 20 weeks the sex can be accurately determined. In reality the sex can be determined earlier by means of ultrasound but this is less accurate. The pregnant mother is measured at each visit to see how the baby's growth is proceeding and the fetus's heart is checked with a fetal Doppler or stethoscope. The weight gain is based on many factors including size of the fetus, volume of the amniotic fluid, and the amount of weight gained by the pregnant mother.

At 28 weeks, hemoglobin is taken to determine if there is anemia of pregnancy, which is fairly common in spite of maternity vitamins. This will often cause tiredness at this stage, and additional supplementation with iron sometimes becomes necessary. There is a new prenatal vitamin available in Canada called PregVit, which I have observed in my practice to lessen the incidence of anemia. It also seems to be better tolerated as far as nausea arising from maternity vitamins.

There are very few remaining tests to do unless other issues crop up during the pregnancy. Further ultrasound exams are sometimes needed; for example, if a baby is suspected of being large or small for its dates, or to establish the position in a baby suspected of being breech (bum first) or transverse lie (lying sideways).

At 35 to 36 weeks one final test is done. An internal vaginal exam shows how low the baby's head is, how well it is applied to the cervix, and whether the cervix is still long or whether it has a central position. All these features are soft predictors of how easy the vaginal delivery is likely to be. Additionally, a simple swab is taken from the recto-vaginal area to establish whether she is carrying bacteria in her vagina known as Group B Strep. Once a pregnant woman goes into labour or ruptures her membranes (breaks her water), there is a possibility that Group B Strep can cause infection to both the mother's uterus as well as to the fetus, resulting in a potentially serious infection. The practice is therefore to start all carriers on intravenous antibiotics four hours after labour begins or once the membranes rupture.

Patients with a history of vaginal herpes are at high risk for passing on the virus during vaginal delivery. As a precaution all these individuals require a prophylactic course of Valtrex®, 500mg twice a day, starting at the 36th week. If at the time of labour, a patient has an outbreak of vaginal/perineal herpes, she will require a C-section in order to deliver the baby.

If at any time during the pregnancy, sugar or protein are shown to be present in the urine, additional tests would then be done to detect gestational diabetes and toxemia of pregnancy. A non-stress test is also sometimes required. This is a measure to see if there is any compromise of the flow *to* the placenta during movement of the baby, or if the baby is compromised due to flow *from* the placenta via the umbilical cord.

Gestational Diabetes

Some women develop gestational diabetes, which if untreated can lead to a larger baby, which can in turn influence the final outcome of the delivery. Delivering a 6 lb baby versus an 8 lb baby can be the influencing factor in how long you might have to push during the second stage, or even the factor resulting in deciding whether to have a natural delivery, an assisted delivery or a C-section.

As a result, at 28 weeks, all women get a one-hour gestational diabetic test and a blood hemoglobin test. The diabetic test involves drinking a 50-gram solution of sugar, which tastes very sweet like Orange Crush. You then have to sit still for an hour, at which point blood is drawn. We have you sit so that you don't burn the sugar faster so that we can get an accurate reading.

If this test is positive, we confirm the results with a similar, but more formal test, the three-hour glucose tolerance test. If this tests confirms gestational diabetes, you will have to see a diabetic specialist who will educate you in diet and manage the diabetes, if necessary through insulin injections.

Hypertension in Pregnancy; Pre-eclampsia (Toxemia)

We can deal with these issues at the same time, starting with hypertension, which is elevated blood pressure. We do our best to lower blood pressure because high blood pressure can cause cerebral hemorrhage and left-ventricular heart failure. It causes a reduction in blood flow to the placenta, which reduces the efficiency of the placenta, which reduces the supply of nourishment to the baby, resulting in a slowing of the growth of the baby. In addition, the ability of the placenta to deal with stress, such as uterine contractions, is also compromised, resulting in the need to deliver the baby sooner.

A resting blood pressure of 140/90 mm Hg or more in the first 24 weeks is unlikely to be due to the pregnancy itself and more likely to be due to the patient having non-pregnancy hypertension. Once any underlying cause such as kidney disease or other medical reason is ruled out, the treatment is rest, a low salt diet, stress reduction, elimination of tannins and caffeine and, finally medication. Methyldopa works well to reduce hypertension in pregnancy and can be given in doses from 500 mg to 4 g daily. Labetalol is another medication effectively used.

Women who start out early in pregnancy with an elevated blood pressure are also at risk of developing further problems such as pre-eclampsia.

Eclampsia is a sudden seizure in pregnancy. It presents with a convulsion and carries very serious consequences as it results in hypoxia or lack of oxygen to the mother and to the baby. It is a serious condition, and the consequences are dependent on the number of seizures, how long they last, and how quickly they can be stopped. Usually this involves using Valium and heavily sedating the patient.

Some women have a pre-syndrome that leads them to develop these seizures. The pre-syndrome is known as pre-eclampsia and is diagnosed in women who are pregnant and have high blood pressure and protein in their urine and excessive weight gain from fluid retention (also known as edema). Pre-eclampsia can also be known as toxemia of pregnancy. For years it was postulated that a toxin was liberated into the system from the pregnant uterus, but we now know that no such toxin exists, thus the term 'Toxemia of pregnancy' is clearly a misnomer.

Pre-eclampsia is a disease of signs, not symptoms, and this is another reason why we are so careful to weigh you, measure your blood pressure and check your urine for protein at each visit. Early diagnosis is crucial.

Pre-eclampsia can evolve very fast, over one day or over a longer period of time, and may have only one sign to begin with. For this reason, hypertension alone, and especially after 24 weeks, should be considered pre-eclampsia until proven otherwise. Realistically pre-eclampsia is found towards the end of the pregnancy. This is one reason why we increase the frequency of visits at 28 weeks to every 2 weeks and at 36 weeks to weekly. The diagnosis of pre-eclampsia is made with additional tests that can indicate a higher risk of developing eclampsia. These are blood tests that include complete blood count (CBC) and a platelet count, liver and kidney function tests, increased regular checking of blood pressure, and of placental function. Placental function can be assessed by a nonstress test (which is discussed) and ultrasound.

The effect of raised blood pressure is to produce damage to the kidneys, liver, placenta, and intestines. More noticeable symptoms emerge as pre-eclampsia advances, such as headaches, epigastric/ heartburn /abdominal pain, and swelling of the legs, feet, ankles, hands and fingers.

The ultimate goal is to allow the pregnancy to advance as close to 37 weeks (term) as possible without compromising either the mother or the baby. The treatment for suspected pre-eclampsia is rest and hospitalization. Further intervention would be to prevent impending seizures with magnesium sulphate and to deliver the baby either via C-section or by vaginal birth. Your obstetrician would determine this after weighing up the pros and cons.

Rhesus Factor

All pregnant women are automatically screened to establish whether they have a protein on the surface of their red blood cells called the Rhesus factor. If they do, they are called Rh-positive. If they do not, they are called Rh-negative.

It is the Rh-negative mother who is a concern. If she is exposed to the blood of her fetus, either because of early bleeding in her pregnancy or later at the time of delivery, this can cause her to produce antibodies against these proteins. This poses a problem for future pregnancies because these antibodies would then attack red blood cells that do have the protein, which would in turn destroy those cells making that fetus anemic. This could potentially result in fetal heart failure in future pregnancies. In developed countries today, this has become a rare condition because we inject all mothers who are Rh-negative with an immunoglobulin called Rhogam. If the fetus is Rh-positive, the Rhogam will bind with any anti-Rh antibodies so that it is eliminated immediately and poses no threat in the future. This shot is given to all Rh-negative mothers at 28 weeks or if they have spotted or bled earlier in the pregnancy. If the newborn is found to be Rh-positive, a further shot is given within 24 hours of childbirth.

Commonly Asked Questions

Weight

Weight gain is a common concern, whether it is about too much or too little weight gained. There are general guidelines, but these fail hopelessly and for the most part cause much anxiety for women. I have adopted a general rule that seems to work well for all: a weight gain of between 15 and 25 lbs over the course of the pregnancy is ideal. Both the Society of Obstetrics and Gynecologists of Canada and the American College of Obstetricians and Gynecologists have suggested that the optimal weight gain should be 15 lbs over the whole pregnancy, but, realistically, I very rarely see this goal achieved. In fact, I would say that the average woman gains between 35 and 40 lbs. As a rule, in the first trimester there is often a very slight weight gain due to the nausea experienced. Sometimes there may even be a slight weight loss. This may be a big concern for the woman, but is often corrected going in to the second trimester at which time her appetite improves.

Most women tend to gain weight consistently from one visit to the next, while others will see a big jump from one visit to the next, but a very small gain over the following few visits. I usually reassure those who gain 7 lbs in 2 weeks that this won't be a regular occurrence. But I also will confirm that the mom is not overdoing the pop and juices, all of which are loaded with calories, and that their diet is conservative, with moderate caloric consumption, and is not filled with junk food.

Sometimes there is a particular cause of the weight gain, such as water retention towards the last trimester and indulgence in foods high in salt. It can also reflect an underlying problem like gestational diabetes, which we have already discussed, or a condition called polyhydramnios where too much amniotic fluid is produced.

Of greater concern is weight loss, which may indicate a problem with weight loss in the baby, also called IUGR or intra-uterine growth retardation, which will often be identified with an ultrasound or a non-stress test. It may reflect that the mother is not eating enough. It may reflect that the baby is not gaining and it could also be a sign that the amniotic fluid has decreased.

One instance of weight loss that is not so much cause for concern is when a patient has a large jump in weight due to water retention and then restricts her salt intake so that on the next visit there is an apparent weight loss, when in fact there is a loss of fluid.

Generally weight loss or gain is assessed in its full context by looking at the whole clinical picture, which is why the height of uterus/fundus is measured with each visit.

Anemia

Anemia is another common issue. In pregnancy, blood is diverted from the mother to the fetus and placenta, providing the placenta and the fetus with the necessary nutrients. For this reason, expectant moms require extra iron intake in their diet so that they can increase their hemoglobin and so that they do not become more fatigued as the pregnancy progresses. This often is only achieved with an addition of oral iron to the prenatal vitamin already being taken.

Miscarriage

Miscarriage is a big concern when a mother comes in with either cramping and or spotting in the first trimester. The first bad sign is when she has period-type cramps and heavy bleeding with or without clots of blood. The miscarriage can be confirmed with an ultrasound. Sometimes, however, an ultrasound can be difficult to obtain in many centres as an outpatient, and in those situations a quantitative b-HCG test can be done for three consecutive days. This test measures the amount of pregnancy hormone in the mother's blood, which increases each day in the first 10 to 11 weeks. At the 11th week this test becomes more difficult to interpret because the level reaches a maximum value and then starts to drop thereafter. An ultrasound will be difficult to interpret if the pregnancy is under 6 weeks and the fetal heart is not seen, because the fetal heart is usually only seen *after* the 6th week. An ultrasound can also be used to illustrate whether this is an ectopic pregnancy, which we discuss in the next section.

Miscarriage is one of those complications seen in one out of five pregnancies. The first thing is to recognize that this occurs regardless of the alcohol consumed prior to finding out about the pregnancy. It has no correlation with how hard you have been working, how stressful life is, how much intercourse you have had since conception.

Sadly, we have created a world of the now factor. We have set ourselves up with our early positive pregnancy tests that tell women that they have conceived ten days after intercourse and even prior to a missed period. In the old days, you missed your period and you put it down to stress. On the second missed period you thought that you might be pregnant, and by the third missed period, things started to show, so now you were sure. But if you miscarried in the middle of all of this, you just had what you thought of as a normal period and you were none the wiser.

Most pregnancies that make it to the twelfth week can be considered viable. If a pregnancy is lost after this, then it is usually uncommon and as a result of the cervix not having the ability to contain the products of the pregnancy within the uterus. This is called an incompetent cervix. Other less common causes of fetal demise and miscarriage after the 12th week include infections in the uterus or amniotic fluid, or complications of the development of the baby, the uterus or the amniotic fluid.

Once the baby has made it to 25 weeks or is larger than 1000 g and should labour begin, the fetus, by definition, becomes viable. This signifies that this is now a viable pregnancy, so if the mother were to go into early labour, or her waters break, this is no longer referred to as a miscarriage, but as preterm labour or premature rupture of the membranes.

Ectopic Pregnancy

This is an uncommon type of pregnancy whereby the fertilized egg does not descend down the fallopian tube to implant into the uterus but instead implants within the tube itself. This type of pregnancy is never successful and can result in serious consequences for the pregnant mother. It may present with abdominal pain and or vaginal bleeding and can result in the bursting of a tube. This is why it is important to diagnose as it can result in hemorrhage. It sometimes presents with shoulder tip pain.

Pain

Pain and its causes probably produce the most anxiety of any of the many new things experienced in pregnancy. For a first-time mother, this pain has never been experienced before, and often she is concerned that there is a problem with the baby. Conversely, a mother who has already experienced pregnancy will have expectations that things should feel the same as in her previous pregnancies, and often they do not.

In the beginning, the first 12 weeks involve a physiological normal growth of the uterus out of the pelvis and into the abdominal cavity. This growth results in a stretching of the uterus and all its surrounding muscles and ligaments. Often this will result in a feeling of cramps. Women often feel that they may be getting their period. There is sometimes a small bit of spotting which adds to the concern. Spotting is usually due to implantation of the placenta and expansion of the placenta within the uterine wall. In addition, there is also increased blood flow and softening of the cervix, and this may be another reason for spotting, especially after intercourse.

After the 12th week, many physiological pains are experienced. The most common initial pains are all related to the initial growth and stretching of the uterus as it grows out of the pelvic cavity. The uterus is supported and suspended on either side, like a suspension bridge, by the round ligaments, rope-like structures that attach to the pelvic wall. As the uterus enlarges and grows, it causes the ligaments to stretch, which places more tension on them. These ligaments keep the uterus in place when a pregnant woman stands and thus prevent a uterus from falling forwards. As we can imagine, this gets tougher as the pregnancy advances. The longer a woman stands, the greater the pain from this stretching process becomes, so that it is more often a problem in women who are in standing jobs.

A diagnosis of round ligament pain may be confirmed with the patient lying down by moving the uterus side to side, causing a tension of the round ligaments. Sometimes it may be just one of these ligaments involved, in which case the pain is only on the one side.

Other pains we see are related to the increasing size of the uterus, which the pelvis and abdomen must accommodate.

In order to accommodate the fetal parts as well as the uterus, the pelvis has to relax. A multitude of hormones and amino acids are released in pregnancy, which cause the ligaments to relax. This is seen especially around the major bones that make up the pelvis, including the sacroiliac joint, the pubic symphysis and the coccyx. This can result in sacroiliac or buttock pain with or without sciatica and also in pain in the centre of the pelvis with sharp shooting pain in the midline of the pelvis.

Further complaints are of lower back pain due to the increased accommodating size of the abdomen and the pressure on the ligaments and muscles of the lower back.

There are several support products that aid in providing extra support for these changing areas to correct or relieve these changes. A product called Mom-Ez is available and is an elastic tensor-type support that acts as a support for a pedunculated protruding abdomen. Correcting this and providing an external harness support brings relief to the lower back and hip area. A similar product is available as a sacroiliac external support to help relieve patients with sacroiliac problems and pain.

Carpal Tunnel Syndrome

This condition is surprisingly common in pregnancy and especially in the last trimester. It is characterized by numbness in the fingers and the hand, mainly in the inner portion of the palm side. This can be worse especially at night and may often awaken the woman. The remedy for getting rid of the numbness is to drop the hand over the side of the bed and massage the hand and wrist.

Carpal tunnel syndrome is caused by retention of fluid that causes swelling around the median nerve. This nerve, which is found in the hand, originates at the wrist and travels through a tunnel in the wrist bones called the carpal tunnel. When the wrist is bent, the tunnel narrows. Usually there is enough space in this tunnel, but when we sleep, *we all* sleep with our wrists bent. When you are pregnant, the conjunction of the bent wrist with the water retention towards the end of your pregnancy results in pressure on the nerve, and thus numbness. Sometimes this is quite a challenge. The best treatment is to have a low salt diet and to wear a Velcro wrist splint while sleeping to avoid bending your wrist. Most patients have complete resolution of this problem after delivery.

Leg Cramps

This is a common complaint and is especially worse later in pregnancy. It is caused by a lack of potassium, calcium and or magnesium in the diet. If this occurs, it can be easily prevented by increasing your potassium intake in the form of bananas and oranges, and by increasing dark green leafy vegetables and low fat dairy products. Supplements with 400 mg magnesium and 800 mg calcium will further prevent this problem.

In the meantime, if you experience a leg cramp, do not panic. It is important to immediately straighten your leg and knee and to pull your big toe upwards towards you. If you do not, then the spasm occurs, causing pain. We tend to do the opposite, relaxing and bending the knee, and this generally makes things worse.

Nasal Stuffiness

Pregnant women often believe that they are coming down with a cold. Increased blood flow to the nasal tissue creates nasal venous congestion, forcing them to breathe through their mouths. A husband will often comment on his new-sounding wife who has given a new meaning to the word snoring. It is difficult to treat, but to preserve the sanity of all involved, nasal sprays such as Otrivin® and/or nasal anti-inflammatories may be used. Nasal strips that are applied over the bridge of the nose may help correct this problem for some. Breathe Right® nasal strips are available in North America.

Hair and Skin Changes

Pregnancy hormones affect many things. Hair changes may occur, with hair growth increasing in areas that usually do not have hair, such as the upper lip, the abdomen, and even the extremities. Similarly, increased pigment may occur such as the mask of pregnancy on the face and the linea alba in the midline of the abdomen. Some women glow in pregnancy and swear that their skin has never looked better. Others develop acne and swear that pregnancy has caused it, and they are so right! The good news for those cursing is that once the pregnancy is over and the hormones are gone, these skin and hair changes disappear too. While on the topic of hair, coloring is not harmful to the baby so if this is something you are thinking of --- go for it.

Heartburn and Acid Reflux

The cause of heartburn and acid reflux is not because of the amount of hair on your baby's head. It is due to the growing uterus and its displacement of the bowel, and in turn the stomach. The stomach has a valve or sphincter; once this is displaced, it does not hold the stomach contents down. Thus acid and food are allowed to regurgitate or reflux up into the esophagus and mouth. This is noted as being a sour acidic taste or as heartburn. Both heartburn and acid reflux may cause lots of grief, and often over-the-counter (OTC) products such as Tums® and other antacids just don't cut it. There are other products safe to take such as the H2 receptor blockers, including such as Zantac 75®, Pepcid® AC, etc. If the OTC products fail, there are further prescription products for further treatment; one example is omeprazole or Losec®.

Other non-drug options to this problem include smaller meals, placement of blocks at the head of the bed so that you are sleeping uphill, thus allowing gravity to work against the reflux.

Additional problems are related to the increase in size of the uterus and the pressure effects on surrounding structures such as the bladder and the bowels.

Pressure on the Bladder

I often hear complaints of frequent urination, due to pressure on the bladder. The solution to this is limited: reduce your intake of fluids at night to reduce your frequency of bathroom visits at night.

Pressure on the Bowel

The effects are seen in the form of constipation and hemorrhoids. Increase your fibre intake in the form of high fibre cereals and high fibre supplements, such as Metamucil® and Prodium®.

Vaginal Discharge

In many women, this is purely due to hormonal changes resulting in an increase in vaginal secretions. For the same reason, there is also an increased chance of developing a yeast infection. The two can be distinguished from one another in that yeast infection tends to cause itching and irritation to the vagina and external perineal tissue, with the discharge often being thicker and clumpier, like cottage cheese. Yeast or fungal infections are treated with conventional anti-fungal topicals in cream or as a pessary, which is a solid tablet that is inserted into the vagina.

Pregnancy hormones increase the amount of normal vaginal secretions causing a discharge called leucorrhoea of pregnancy. It is often misinterpreted as a bladder infection, because the urine becomes contaminated with the discharge when you urinate, resulting in cloudiness in the urine. The urine may also show pus cells that are in fact from this vaginal discharge. For this reason, when I do a routine urinalysis to check protein and sugar in your regular visits, I do not routinely include a urinary white cell test, because it always tests positive.

Leg swelling

Many women experience leg swelling in pregnancy. As the pregnancy advances, the tendency is for this to become worse, commonly resulting in more discomfort and limitation in mobility as well as a need for comfortable footwear.

Many causes contribute to this problem: how long you are on your feet, the amount of your salt intake, as well as many other factors. Pregnant women are specifically affected because the pregnancy hormones relax the muscle walls of these veins, and as a result of this relaxed tone, the veins fail to pump blood efficiently back to the heart. Blood pools in the legs, causing swelling of the soft tissue.

To reduce swollen feet, you should try and reduce the time you spend standing, elevate your feet, cut out all salts hidden in food and drink, and rule out any medical causes such as high blood pressure. Another very useful aid is a pair of good support stockings to be worn during the day and to provide external support to the veins in the legs. The Samson & Delilah series of support hose, made by Sigvaris, is a good over-the-counter stocking.

Varicose Veins

The same factors that produce leg swelling also result in varicose veins, except that the veins affected are those found on the surface and not the deep ones. Varicose veins may cause discomfort and itching. If they are very small, they may cause cosmetically unsightly veins. The treatment is the same as for leg swelling, but the veins may remain after the pregnancy, in which case they may require further treatment.

Sex During Pregnancy

Pregnancy will result in a change in hormones, which in turn will cause a different response in each individual. The response I am referring to is sexual desire or libido.

There are other contributing factors in the initial stages of pregnancy such as how sick you may feel and how much energy you have. For many women, intercourse is the furthest thing from their minds, what with all their throwing up and sleeping. For others, they are so sexually aroused that they are worried about this change in themselves. There is also a fear that intercourse may hurt the baby or cause a miscarriage.

There are only a few scenarios that may result in a limit on intercourse, such as an infection of the uterus or amniotic fluid, a bladder infection, bleeding, or a problem with the placenta being in the lower uterus lying over the cervix (also known as placenta praevia). The last example occurs in women who have broken their waters or amniotic fluid.

A limit on intercourse does not necessarily restrict a couple from intimacy or lovemaking, which can be just as enjoyable, especially for women whose breast and vaginal sensitivity is increased by hormones.

Sex is not only safe, but it should be less stressful as no birth control is required.

Travel

There is no harm to the baby in traveling at any time during pregnancy whether by air or sea. Your travel company is concerned about how likely you are to go into labour, which then becomes a liability for the travel carrier. Many air-carriers do not allow travel if a woman is over 36 weeks pregnant. Good medical coverage becomes important especially when traveling out of country.

Flu Shots and Other Immunizations

The flu shot is safe in pregnancy and is often advocated in the last trimester as it provides the mother with immunity and prevents her from passing any viral influenza to her newborn infant.

Any one of the live-attenuated immunizations, such as rubella, measles, mumps and chickenpox, are considered contraindicated in pregnancy. These vaccines are live but not infectious like the wild form, rendering them unsafe during pregnancy.

Fetal Movement

If this is your first pregnancy, fetal movement is usually felt at about 23 weeks and may be confused with a feeling of gas in the lower abdominal area. Fetal movement or quickening may be felt earlier in subsequent pregnancies—often as early as 16 weeks. Movement is sometimes quite vigorous at certain times of the day. Often women are concerned that the baby may be having a convulsion because they feel a repetitive movement. This is, in fact, hiccups and is perfectly normal.

Body parts are quite easy to feel and to make out at about 32 weeks. This is usually impossible at 28 weeks and earlier.

After 32 weeks, it is a good practice to establish what time of day your baby is most active. Once you have identified this, you can establish a routine of doing a fetal movement count every week at this active time. During its most active time, the baby should move at least 4 times an hour. This is then considered a normal count.

Membrane stripping

This is a process by which a doctor or midwife does a vaginal exam and places his or her finger within the cervix and strips the amniotic membranes. It is a practice that is supposed to initiate labour. It is not a procedure that I perform, however, as I am concerned that by causing trauma to the membranes one can cause the amniotic fluid to leak. This is comparable to piercing a balloon filled with water. The pressure of the water will expand the hole, causing the balloon to break. The problem here is that if the baby's presenting part is high above the cervix, the cord can potentially drop down ahead of the baby.

This is a very serious problem and can result in fetal death. By stripping membranes, you are also at risk of causing infection in the amniotic fluid and this can cause the mother and the baby to become septic. It is for this reason I believe that if you wish to induce labour, it must be done in another more formal way such as with prostaglandin gel, Cervidil®, or with oxytocin.

Dispelling the Myths of Pregnancy

There are so many mythical beliefs around the topic of pregnancy. I hope that this section will clarify some of them for you.

Sex of the Baby

Can you determine the sex of the baby ahead of time? The answer is yes. This may be determined by means of chromosomal analysis by amniocentesis, or by doing an ultrasound examination at twenty weeks. Ultrasound may be less reliable as there are more variants to the process, such as maternal size, fetal position, kind of ultrasound machine, and experience of the technician.

Fetal heart rate is never a determining factor. There have been occasions when pregnant women have been told that fetal heart rate is indeed a determining factor, even by health care professionals. It truly makes no sense as heart rate goes up with activity and goes down with rest. This is the same phenomenon that occurs in adults when they exercise or relax. And adults certainly don't change sex with heart rate fluctuations!

The myth lives on, however, as there is a 50:50 chance of a correct determination. This explains why the Aunt Bettys of the world who have correctly predicted the sex in each of the family's last 30 births will occasionally have a bad day and read the heart rate predictors incorrectly. I don't think so!

Fetal heart rate varies between 120 and 160 beats per minute.

At the beginning of the pregnancy, the heart rate tends to be faster at 160 beats per minute. As the fetus matures over the course of the pregnancy, the fetal heart rate tends to slow down to a slower rate of around 120 beats per minute. During a prenatal visit, the heart rate may increase with fetal activity and decrease when the fetus is sleeping.

All other tests such as the tealeaf test, the hair test, etc., should be ignored.

The next poor determinant is that of size and sex of the baby based on 'the way you carry'. This is something noted in malls and elevators by so-called experts who will gladly provide an assessment, at no cost to you, and of absolutely no value to you either.

'The Way You Carry'

The term 'the way you carry' is a description of the pedunculous girth of the abdomen of a pregnant patient. Doctors and midwives never examine a pregnant woman when she is standing up because nothing can be determined by examining her in this position. But when a pregnant woman lies on her back, the top of the uterus can be felt through the abdominal muscles, and thus the uterus can be measured from the pelvis to the top of the uterus. This is the most accurate measure of the fetal size. When a woman is standing, the factors that may make her look larger and affect 'the way she carries' are the following: the strength of the abdominal muscles, the laxity of the round ligaments, the amount of amniotic fluid, and the posture of the patient. All these factors hugely determine how one looks. So often a patient looks huge, and once she lies down, the uterus is found to be normal. Sometimes the concerned relatives will send a mother in because they feel the baby is too small. This is often a young woman with no abdominal fat, but solid anterior abdominal muscles that hold the abdominal contents contained.

Size of the Baby

Another huge myth is the divine knowledge of how big the baby is. In all honesty, I do not know any doctor or health provider who *truly* knows the size of the baby by clinical exam. This is a blind science. What we do know is that there is a baby in the uterus of unknown size, surrounded by amniotic fluid of unknown quantity. This is what makes it so difficult. The best analogy is to take two turkeys, one 6 lb and one 9 lb. Place each in a black garbage bag filled with 3 litres of water and tie the bags. It is impossible to tell which bag contains the larger turkey.

I had a humbling experience when I attended a C-section with one of my distinguished obstetrical colleagues who was nearing retirement and whose opinion I truly valued. As he was speaking to the patient, she turned to him, indicating that *I* wouldn't know but that *he* would be able to tell how large her baby was. He agreed and proceeded to examine her pregnant belly with much authority. He hummed and ha-ed, and frowned and pouted and then as his brain drew on its years of valuable expertise he declared that this baby would be about 9 lbs. Well, this C-sectioned baby must have shrunk somewhere between its delivery in the operating room and the nursery scale as it weighed in at about 6 lbs. This vivid encounter again confirmed the truth of the old turkey-in-the-bag story that I like to tell my pregnant patients.

When is the Baby Due?

My generic advice is to take the due date that you have been given and to add 10 days to this. Then give this date out to all your friends and family. The reason for adding ten days is that this would be the time when we would induce labour because at that point there is no further benefit to being pregnant. The baby is as mature as it can get, and the placenta starts to calcify as it is over-matured and cannot sustain the baby.

This date calculation thus prevents the inevitable stress that begins once the due date has come and gone, and all the calls start to come in. And with the calls, comes the mythical advice on how to go into labour. Human nature makes us rationalize that because a term baby is a baby over 36 weeks, that baby can come any time after 36 weeks. Interestingly, most women go over their due date, and more women get induced than actually have their babies before their due date.

Fetal Parts

I am often asked to point out the fetal parts, which is often a challenge. This is something that is often determined by so many factors such as the amount of amniotic fluid, the size of the baby, and the amount of fat covering the abdomen of the expectant mother. Often, fetal parts can be seen sporadically from 26 weeks and up, but tend to be a lot easier to identify and point out at 32 to 34 weeks.

Predictive Measures

There are a bunch of things that are looked at and interpreted as a *sign* of things about to happen—like labour. For example, if the baby drops, does this mean that labour is going to follow soon? Or would a vaginal exam predict when labour would begin?

There used to be a predictive score that has since proven to be unreliable. Bishop's score was performed at 36 weeks, and 2 points were allotted for each finding at this exam. It looked at things such as pelvic measurements, the location of the baby's head in relation to the pelvis, and the position and thickness of the cervix.

It is also now recognized that it is impossible in almost every instance to predict in advance the likeliness of vaginal birth. Every woman should be allowed the opportunity for normal childbirth—what we call a fair trial of labour. It is impossible to look at a key in relation to a lock and in advance to know whether the key will fit and be able to open the lock.

There are several books that place much importance on whether the baby has dropped and this is seen as an indicator of impending labour. I beg to differ. I have never found this to be a reliable indicator of whether labour is about to begin.

In my opinion, labour begins when a switch within the pituitary gland is turned on. This in turn releases oxytocin, which causes uterine contractions.

Another sign that is also unpredictable is something called a 'show'. This is where a vaginal discharge occurs with a mucous component. Sometimes a bit of blood may also be seen. This show is supposed to appear prior to going into labour. It is usually a mucous plug that originates from the cervix and is released as the cervix softens in the last month. Many times a patient will lose the plug and come in quite upset that she has not gone into labour. Labour is often the next thing to occur after a show, but this can take as long as two to four weeks.

Preterm Labour

Preterm labour is labour that begins three or more weeks before the due date. It is also seen as labour that starts at 37 weeks or less. Because the labour begins early, it makes sense that the baby is born earlier, making it a premature baby.

Sometimes preterm labour occurs for unknown reasons. Certain factors are known, however, to increase a women's risk of preterm labour. These include:

♦ multiple pregnancies, such as twins or more
♦ previous preterm baby
♦ early cervical changes
♦ polyhydramnios (too much amniotic fluid)
♦ smoking
♦ drug abuse such as cocaine
♦ other pregnancy problems such as bleeding or infection
♦ preterm rupture of membranes
♦ mother is less than 17 yrs old

In preterm labour, if the pregnancy is more than 34 weeks, we usually allow the labour to continue. If the pregnancy is less than 34 weeks, the aim is to buy extra time until the baby is 34 weeks or more. We do this by reducing and therefore stopping contractions, and our most valuable tool is rest.

Doctors also use certain medication to slow down labour. Other medications such as corticosteroids can be given to the mother to mature the baby's lungs so that if we do fail to slow down the contractions, if the baby is then born, it at least has more protection against premature lungs.

The corticosteroids mature the lungs in a 24-to-48-hour period, and this can result in the baby having enough of a substance in the lung tissue called surfactant, which will allow the immature lungs to mature and function without the need of a ventilator.

Premature babies are at a higher risk of experiencing problems with breathing, eating and keeping warm. If the baby is born early, it will be smaller and may have underdeveloped lungs. These babies may need care in a special nursery.

Diagnosis and treatment of preterm labour comes with a history from the patient. Signs and symptoms include: uterine tightening or contractions that occur in a cyclical manner and may occur as infrequently as every 10 to 20 minutes, or more often than this. Tightenings are non-painful contractions. They are important warning signs of preterm labour and can be counted by lying down and relaxing your head so that your abdomen is soft. Place your fingertips on the top of your uterus. If the uterus is tightening or contracting, you will feel the abdomen getting tight or hard, and then it will relax again once the contraction or tightening is over. Record the number over an hour. You can also calculate how many minutes go by from the beginning of one to the beginning of the next. You can also time how long the tightening lasts. This can be done over a one-hour period. Other signs are menstrual-like cramps felt in the lower abdomen, which may come and go; pelvic pressure often described as feeling as if the baby is pushing down, which may come and go; bowel cramping with or without diarrhea; bleeding or spotting; increase or change in vaginal discharge. There may be more discharge than usual, or it may change into a mucous-like, watery or light bloody discharge. A sudden gush of fluid from the vagina may mean that the amniotic sac has broken (rupture of membranes).

The most effective treatment of preterm labour is rest. Further investigations in establishing whether you are in preterm labour and how this is affecting the baby are available in the form of a test called a non-stress test. This test monitors the fetal heart rate at the same time as it measures any uterine activity. This is very easy to do by placing one Doppler pick-up to the abdominal wall and another to monitor uterine tightening. Depending on the findings, this test may take between 10 and 60 minutes.

An ultrasound may sometimes be useful to determine if there is any change to the cervix and to look at other factors that may be seen in the baby, the amniotic fluid and placenta that might help better understand and manage the preterm labour.

Premature Rupture of Membranes (PROM)

This term is used when the membrane that forms a sac around the baby breaks before the 37th week of pregnancy.

The fluid within the sac is called amniotic fluid and provides a cushion for the growing baby. The unbroken membranes help to protect the mother and the baby from infection by providing a barrier. When the membrane breaks, the amniotic fluid is released with either a gush or a slow, uncontrollable trickle from the vagina. This fluid continues to be made by the baby's kidneys and lungs so ongoing fluid loss is to be expected until birth.

The cause of premature rupture of membranes is often unknown, but there are several factors that may increase its likelihood. They include: multiple pregnancy (twins, triplets); polyhydramnios (too much amniotic fluid); uterine anomalies; early cervical changes (incompetent cervix); possible infection in the urinary or reproductive tracts.

The aim of treating women with premature rupture of membranes is to minimize the chance of infection and to prolong the pregnancy until the baby is mature (34 to 35) weeks.

So how does this affect the baby?

Premature rupture of membranes may result in labour, contractions and birth. Premature babies have all the problems discussed previously, but with the addition of premature rupture of membranes, there is an additional concern over infection. For this reason, antibiotics are begun automatically in membrane rupture in pregnancies of less than 37 weeks.

If too much amniotic fluid is lost, the cushioning effect provided to the baby is less, and the baby no longer has the same amount of room to freely move around. This can result in the baby's feet being held in an unnatural position. Some babies may need physiotherapy after birth to correct this.

The treatment of PROM is quite similar to that of preterm labour. Indeed, they often go hand in hand, with one often following the other. The principles of treatment are thus quite alike. The most important treatment is rest. The next is to establish if there is infection, by blood tests and monitoring temperature. Further tests such as a non-stress test give us extra information to see how distressed the baby is and if there are any signs of preterm labour associated. Ultrasound can determine how much amniotic fluid has been lost.

Daily checks are done to see if the leaking has slowed down or stopped. The amount of fluid draining is often determined by looking at how many pads are changed per day.

Restrictions include no tub baths, no douching and no intercourse. Other treatment often includes antibiotics and corticosteroids to mature the baby's lungs, especially if the leaking is worsening and contractions or preterm labour begin.

Antepartum Hemorrhage

Bleeding in pregnancy may be seen as a result of many causes. We have already discussed early bleeding due to miscarriage, placental implantation and cervical friability. We now turn to more serious problems.

Antepartum hemorrhage is defined as bleeding from the vagina that occurs at any time after the 28th week of pregnancy and before the birth of the child. This may be divided into 3 categories:

The first category of antepartum hemorrhage is bleeding due to the partial separation of a placenta normally situated on the upper segment of the uterus. This is called accidental hemorrhage, or abruptio placenta. In these cases pregnancy and labour may progress without further bleeding. The term 'accidental hemorrhage' does not refer to trauma, but trauma can be one of the many causes.

The severity of partial separation can vary in nature and result in a considerable variety of symptoms, treatments and final outcomes. It starts with bleeding in some and is characterized in most by a persistent abdominal pain that unlike labour does not come and go.

For example if a patient develops a small bleed behind the placenta and this stops, it may cause pain in the top part of the uterus and there may be very little or no blood. This will usually proceed to a normal delivery. If there is a large amount of blood loss, the separation is more widespread and serious, and the final outcome is more urgent because if the hemorrhage continues, an emergency

C-section becomes necessary. The survival of the baby is more questionable.

Sometimes there can be a large amount of blood loss, and the woman is in shock, but there is very little blood visible, as it remains within the uterine cavity. This is called a concealed hemorrhage. When the blood tracks down between membranes and the wall of the uterus, it escapes into the vagina and is a revealed hemorrhage.

Causes of abruptio placenta include hypertension, pre-eclampsia, chronic nephritis, cocaine abuse, and finally trauma. The outcome depends on how much blood is lost and badly shocked the mother is .The prognosis for the child is bad with a mortality rate of over 50%.

Diagnosis is made by ultrasound and certain blood tests that may reveal even a small bleed.

The second category of antepartum hemorrhage is bleeding due to a partial separation of the placenta abnormally situated on the lower uterine segment. This is called placenta praevia.

In this category, hemorrhage is sometimes inevitable when the lower segment starts to change with uterine growth and especially once labour begins. The bleeding is often unavoidable because of the location of the placenta.

It is classified into four different types. Type 1 is the least serious. The placenta is only partly attached to the lower segment. The lower margin dips into the lower segment but is at a distance from the internal opening of the cervix called the internal os. In Type 2, the placental margin reaches the internal os. In Types 3 & 4, the placenta partly and fully covers the internal os respectively.

This problem is diagnosed ahead of time because this is what we look for on routine ultrasound. The majority of cases are Type 1 in nature and most of these do not pose any problem. As the uterus continues to grow from the time the low placenta is seen, at 18 to

20 weeks, the placenta moves in its location relative to the os. At 32 to 34 weeks, when a follow-up ultrasound is done, the placenta is no longer considered low. The other three types remain low and are an indication that a C-section will be required.

The third category of antepartum hemorrhage is bleeding due to a lesion of the cervix or vagina such as an erosion , a polyp or carcinoma. This may be called incidental hemorrhage.

The Final Days

So you've been to your doctor and you are now 36 weeks pregnant. The internal check up is done, and he tells you that the baby is head down and that any day now you can go into labour and have a baby.

You might take this as he knows something that you don't—that your labour will begin some time soon. This is probably the biggest misconception and biggest frustration that I have seen in pregnant women—the persistent misunderstanding that the doctor knows something that the woman doesn't. The truth is that your doctor knows nothing more than you know unless he has some divine power. And I can assure you that he doesn't. So why does he say this to you? Well, really what he is telling you is that if you do go into labour at this stage, it would be considered normal term labour. In other words, your baby is 36 weeks or more; so other than gaining weight at this point your baby is just sitting and waiting for that little switch that we discussed before to turn on.

And you are now cocooning and getting things ready, and the calls start to come in because you have decided that you probably will go early, but day-to-day you are still waiting in anticipation.

You start to get some contractions that are painful and uncomfortable, and you think that this is it—and within two hours your pains have disappeared. It's what we refer to as false labour. One can distinguish this pain from Braxton-Hicks pain in that Braxton-Hicks is usually not uncomfortable.

This is an extremely frustrating time because at this stage pregnant women are so uncomfortable that they want the doctor to intervene to get the baby out and do anything so that they can go into labour. It's when all the other inducements start coming into place for example, enemas, castor oil, having sex, drinking alcohol, going on a horse ride, etc.

In all honesty, I truly have not found that magical activity or food that will cause a patient to go into labour. If I had found it, I would not be writing this book. I would have patented the product and put it on the shelves for every pregnant woman to take.

This is the time to consider what is ahead: no matter how uncomfortable you are now and no matter how difficult it is for you to get enough sleep, it is nothing compared with the amount of sleep that you won't get once the baby is born. This is the time to enjoy your special moments with your partner (or on your own) because everything is about to change once the baby is born. This is the time to say goodbye to an old chapter in your life and to look forward to a new one. This is the time to enjoy your existing children (if you have any) because after the baby is born, your focus shifts and, the dynamics of your family will, unfortunately, never be the same again.

As the final days approach, a common question is which sleeping position is best. Many women have read somewhere that if you lie on your back you can harm your baby.

So far, I have not yet seen this in my practice. There is no doubt, however, that women with certain problems of intrauterine growth retardation may maximize the flow to the placenta by sleeping on their side. These patients would need to be monitored closely anyway and would need weekly or bi-weekly non-stress tests in which an external fetal heart monitor as well as a uterine biometric monitor is used to determine whether the heart rate of the baby is reactive to the baby's movement and/or to any contractions, namely Braxton-Hicks contractions.

A non-stress test is one measure by which we can see if there is any compromise to the flow of the placenta during the movement of the baby. This occurs if there is less blood being delivered from the placenta to the baby via the umbilical cord. Other measures such as Doppler ultrasound of the cord would also measure a decreased flow.

So, getting back to the issue of whether you can or cannot sleep on your back, go ahead, enjoy it, unless you have been told that your baby is compromised. I believe that the whole confusion of how safe it is to lie on your back originates from a problem that we see in labour where there is a slowing down of the fetal heart during labour that is remedied by placing the woman on her side in order to increase the flow of blood to the baby. This is a different situation entirely.

Birthing Plan

The questions that you should be asking your doctor at this point relate to the actual event of childbirth. First and foremost try and recognize that the term 'birth plan' is a poor one because we truly cannot plan how labour and delivery are going to go.

I often compare labour to a rollercoaster ride. You start off at the beginning with lots of anxiety and as you are about to hop on to the rollercoaster, you can hear screams above you. Once people get off the rollercoaster ride, they generally seem very happy with the end results.

This rollercoaster ride is different to any other rollercoaster ride you have ever been on—because no matter how many times you take the ride, it is never the same. When you get to the top of the hill you realize there are 15 different tracks.

The first track is what we could call an easy ride track. It looks scary, but once you actually ride it, you realize that it is slow, it is easy, and you get to the end, and you go, "Wow! That's all there is?" The other extreme is that you start out slow and you do a loop-de-loop, triple back-somersault flip and end up getting off this one and after cussing, saying you'll never do it again! These are the extremes that you should be prepared for. Anyone who tells you that birth is a walk in the park is lying. That said and done, there are some women who have it comparatively very, very easy. They are the envy of the baby club.

So now that you are all prepared, what can you expect? Only

one of two things. The first, and the most common, is that you will go into labour. The other possibility on the big day is that labour does not ensue, but that you have spontaneous rupture of membranes prior to any contractions.

Spontaneous Rupture of Membranes

In a situation like this, I generally recommend that you observe the colour of the ruptured amniotic fluid. If it is reasonably clear, there is no major concern. If it is discoloured and green or yellow, it generally indicates that the baby has pooped inside the amniotic fluid—this is called meconium. Usually, it has little significance, but in some instances it could indicate that there is some degree of fetal distress.

Whether the amniotic fluid is clear or discoloured, my general rule is to assess you fairly soon after this happens. Often this requires an external fetal monitor and myometrical measurement of the uterus to see if there are early contractions. If active labour does not begin after 24 hours, the plan is to induce labour because of the prolonged rupture of membranes. We will discuss augmentation of labour whereby intravenous oxytocin is administered to increase the contractions.

If you are not in labour, however, but your membranes have ruptured, a more natural approach is to apply prostaglandin gel (Prostin® E2), which will initiate uterine contractions in almost exactly the same way as labour does. The gel can be applied every 12 hours, so if the gel does not bring on labour within 12 hours, a second and possibly even a third application can be administered. A newer, longer-acting prostaglandin called Cervidil is recently gaining favour in some centres because it is inserted behind the cervix. It needs to be given every 24 hours and works the same way as a 12-hour prostaglandin to start contractions.

For a woman who has advanced 10 days beyond her due date—where this has been confirmed by both calculation of the first day of her last menstrual period and a reliable ultrasound—an induction is indicated, as she is post-dates.

Studies have demonstrated over many years in multiple trials and in many centres that there is no advantage to induction in a woman who wishes to be induced simply because it is convenient for her. In fact, the C-section rate quite significantly increases when induction is done as a convenience to the woman. Feeling too big, or being tired of being pregnant, or having a doctor who is going on holiday, are all issues of convenience. Criteria such as these should not be taken as a need for induction in British Columbia, and in most larger centres in Canada with good clinical practice in obstetrics, because this will increase the frequency and the chance of complications.

If a woman should go 10 days past her due date, there is a significant increase in fetal distress, as well as morbidity and mortality due to the aging placenta. The key time to induce, therefore, without increasing the risk of C-section is at the 10th day beyond the due date.

Preventative antibiotics are given in all those who have been identified as positive for Group B strep. Prophylactic antibiotics would also be indicated in women who are negative for Group B strep but with premature labour at less than 37 weeks.

Statistically most women will go over their due date. More women are induced than go into labour before their due date. In fact, in my practice, I would submit that most women go over their due date, and that as many as 1 in 5 women (20 percent) will need induction. I would also say that only about 5 to 10 percent of women go into labour before their due date.

I also note that history usually repeats itself. If your circumstances are for the most part the same (you have the same partner, and not too much time has lapsed between pregnancies), you will deliver at about the same time as in your previous pregnancy.

How Do You Know if You Are in Labour?

You will start to get contractions either in the front of your abdomen or in your back depending on the position of the baby. Back labour can sometimes be difficult to figure out. The key is to actually look at the definition of labour, i.e., a uterine contraction that is followed by a sequence of contractions, which occur in increasing frequency, duration and intensity.

Labour can be divided into three stages. The first stage is when contractions first begin. The second stage is the pushing, and the third stage is the final part when the placenta is delivered.

Labour is tough enough that in those parts of the world where they celebrate Labour Day, they really should be celebrating the labour of childbirth. It's so tough it requires a public holiday!

I am sure that you have perhaps heard of a woman who was in labour for five days. She truly could not have been in labour for five days because this would not be possible. The most likely situation is that she was in what is called the latent phase of labour in which she gets labour pain that *occurs* at a certain frequency, duration, and intensity, but does not *increase* in frequency, duration, and intensity. In order for labour to progress from the latent phase to the active phase, this increase in frequency, duration, and intensity must occur.

I often liken the latent phase of labour to an older man cranking a motor that will allow the curtain in front of a movie screen to open. Once the movie begins, we will consider this to be the beginning of second stage of labour. This is the time for the woman to begin pushing. So in order to get to this stage, we have to go through the first stage of labour, which is divided into the latent and active phases. Getting back to the old fellow, if he doesn't have the physical power to crank the curtain so that the curtains open fully, the movie cannot begin. This power is necessary to create an opening of the cervix from 0 to 10 cm.

Attempts to push the baby out before the cervix is fully dilated to 10 cm would cause a delay in the second stage of labour. You cannot therefore push until you are fully dilated to 10 cm.

Let's get back to our old fellow. If he keeps cranking the motor but he really doesn't have any power to do it, the curtains can stay open at 2 cm and never progress to 10 cm. If he keeps falling asleep on the job, then he doesn't create any momentum whatsoever. This would be the typical example of the latent phase of labour.

But if we replace him with a big strapping lifeguard-type of guy, who cranks with increasing frequency, intensity and duration, the curtain in front of the screen opens. Full dilation is now achieved.

There is usually a direct correlation between the severity and intensity of the labour and how fast the woman will progress, but this is not always the case. We have mentioned a previous assessment called Bishop's score, which used to predict when labour would begin, but there were even older measurements for determining how successful a woman would be in having a baby. There was a time where X-ray pelvimetry, ultrasound, and manual measurements of the pelvis would give us an idea as to what the outcome of labour would be. Unfortunately, these are all futile in the big picture.

The reason is that you can look at a key and lock and try and be subjective or even objective about whether the key will fit, but the only definitive way of knowing is to do a functional assessment—turn the key in the lock.

Remember that labour is a dynamic process: it occurs with the opening of the cervix in the first stage and of pushing in the second stage, so that the baby can go down the birth canal. If the baby's head is tiny, but in a rotated position facing the wrong way or in a deflexed position, then the relative circumference of the head to the pelvic inlet and outlet can vary. It is this variation that results in a failure to progress in the first and/or second stages of labour, which results in some form of intervention.

Once a patient has reached the active part of labour, she has progressed from 0 to 3 cm, and this often signifies the start of pain requiring intervention.

Water Births

This topic often makes me want to crack up. All right—I know what you are thinking. You are saying that this is very judgmental. How dare he have such a closed mind! But just hear me out on this one.

I am often asked in all sincerity about this as an option for childbirth. And I have seen the videos. The rationale for water birth advocates that the baby who has floated in a pool of amniotic fluid for the past 40 weeks should now be born into another body of fluid.

Supposedly, the whole process is almost natural and most pleasant for the baby. Furthermore, it is supposed to result in less pain for the expectant mother. This is not the case!

Okay, here is the problem. Monitored care is the reason for the current reduced infant-maternal mortality and morbidity rate in the year 2006 in developed countries. This means that at specific points during the first and second stages of labour, we monitor the fetal heart and assess how the baby is doing. We look for changes in the baby's heart rate and its response to the contractions and to pushing. This becomes impossible when you are immersed in a pool of water.

And I also wonder how long you would wish to remain in the water before it becomes cold (unless it is continuously reheated) or you start to wrinkle up like a prune.

Finally, what is the point? For pain control? If I am in a hot tub and I am passing a kidney stone, does this mean that my pain will go? If that were the case, every emergency room would be equipped with a hot tub for anyone passing a kidney stone. So, in reality, the pain might be a little less, but overall, not by a whole lot.

What about making it easier on the baby? Well why? The baby is not a fish or amphibian. It is human. Humans live on land, not in water. We are designed to have babies on dry land. And guess what ... babies are designed to take their first breath on land. If they don't, and they are born into water and the cord is clamped, they have no means of getting oxygen—because they do not have gills at birth. So, once born in water, they would have to come onto dry land anyway to take their first breath, which is ultimately what happens for all births without running the risk of not being able to monitor the baby.

Part of the process of resuscitation in a newborn is to dry, suction, and heat. All of these things are impossible to do in water.

I guess the whole concept is somewhat of a fantasy—almost like having sex in water—it is way overrated.

A few of the more trivial but pertinent concerns are the issues of shaving and enemas.

Shaving does not happen unless you are going for a C-section, and even then it depends on the surgeon. Enemas are not given any more.

Pain and Labour

It often amazes me how impossible it is to predict who is going to need drug intervention and who is not. First of all it is important to know that no one should be empowered to judge you for the pain that you are about to experience in labour—be it bad or be it not. I have seen women who have told me at the onset that they are big sissies and that there is no way they can endure any form of pain. They have gone on to shock both themselves and their family by having no pain intervention whatsoever during their labour.

Then there are women who are the super-athlete, macho, big-muscled type, who've had root canals without any pain medication. But once they go into labour, they yell and scream like anyone. So I always tell women to go into this with an open mind, *and* to know all the possible interventions. I know that if I were to have a kidney stone and I was in the ER, under no circumstances would I accept conservative treatment as an option. I would demand something for pain.

I like to remind women that the first stage of labour can be tedious. I tell them about the latent and active phases in the first stage of labour, and I emphasize that patients should recognize that all the work really begins at the second stage of labour. This is when the woman needs to push. Pushing, especially if this is your first baby, can require a full two hours, and then some, to push the baby out. So try to get as much help as possible in the first stage of labour, so that when the second stage of labour comes, you are re-energized and have two hours of energy to spare.

The most frustrating part for you will be to reach dilation of 10 cm and then be asked to push, only to realize that you are too tired. At this point, I have nothing to offer you, because it is finally up to you to start pushing.

So, now you have arrived, and you want something for pain because you are 3 cm dilated, what are your options? Non-drug options are often a woman's first choice. These include heat or water, massage, aromatherapy, meditation, pressure point kinesiology, acupuncture, and hypnosis. If any of these work for you as a first option, that's great. If not, we move on to the drug options.

The first is Entanox, also known as nitrous oxide gas or laughing gas. It is breathed in through a mask or a mouthpiece and immediately (after just two or three breaths) causes some degree of relaxation and relief. Women often liken this to feeling a little bit drunk and giddy in their heads. As a general rule if women are okay with feeling like this, they do very well with the gas. If this makes them feel out of control, then they often prefer to try something else. This is the simplest form of pain intervention, however, and is worth a try. It generally wears off within a couple minutes of no longer breathing it in, and it can be administered right throughout the first and second stages of labour. There is no negative effect on the baby. You might find it tiring, however, to keep on sucking gas for hours.

The next possibility is to use narcotics. In Canada, the two options are Demerol® and Fentanyl. Demerol is usually given intramuscularly but can be given by other methods as well. When given intramuscularly it can last up to three to four hours. There are some restrictions as to when these drugs can be administered. For example, Demerol is not given at the beginning of labour as it can push the woman out of labour when given too early. It also should not be given too late, as it is a narcotic and will sedate the woman. If Demerol is given when the woman is dilated more than 8 cm, when it is time to push, especially if things progress rapidly, she may be too mentally impaired to cooperate in terms of pushing.

Another concern is that upon delivery the baby would be too sedated if Demerol were still circulating in the mother's blood, leading to compromise of the baby's respiratory system at birth.

Fentanyl is administered intravenously. It cannot be given to a woman who is either under or overweight, but it can be administered to the average woman at the end stages, as it is absorbed and broken down within 30 minutes—much more quickly than Demerol. It can thus be given as a bridge in the last hour of labour and is often used when Demerol is contraindicated and where it is just buying an extra 30 minutes of time before the woman starts to push. The ideal time that this can be useful is during transition. This is a time during the first stage when the woman reaches a point where the pain is extreme, she feels weak in her knees, and she starts to shake without any control. She is usually at about 7 to 8 cm dilation when this occurs.

Your last option is an epidural. Time and time again, when you read about epidurals, they are a no-no, as there are major complications that can supposedly occur as a result. The word 'epidural' is an abbreviation of the term given to a procedure where numerous drugs are injected into the epidural space inside the bones of the back, but outside the spinal fluid. Nerves travel through this space just before collecting together to form the spinal cord. This space turns out to be a good place to put drugs, as it allows both sides of the body to be frozen with one injection. Also the space is big enough to insert a small plastic tube, which allows a continuous flow of anesthetic drugs to keep you comfortable over the time of labour. The amount of drug that potentially gets to the baby is negligible.

The drugs given into the epidural space are often a cocktail of local anesthetic, namely bupivicaine and ropivacaine. Fentanyl also forms part of this cocktail. Depending on the different strengths and combinations, we see different end results in the effect of the epidural. A 'walking' epidural is one example. A woman gets the benefits of pain relief and can continue to move her legs, allowing her to walk. In reality this is difficult to do in that once you have an epidural your blood pressure drops and you do need close monitoring so that walking with an epidural becomes impractical.

In my experience, I have rarely heard a woman complain that she hates the epidural. Usually she hugs the anesthetist administering the epidural and is forever thankful to him.

Sometimes, we see a post-epidural headache, and more rarely we will see other complications from an epidural. For example, when the needle pierces through both sides of the epidural lining producing a more substantial headache, or one of the blood vessels is pierced, resulting in more substantial localized pain in the location of the epidural. Other than that, epidurals are well tolerated and facilitate many women in labour.

One of the drawbacks of an epidural is that if you give it too early, it can result in a slowing down of the contractions, and if you give it too late—when the woman is 8 to 9 cm dilated—it can result in the woman not having any sensation. She is unable to focus where she is pushing, which causes a delay in the initiation of the second stage of labour. In reality an epidural can be given at any time but practically it may complicate things. Once the woman reaches her second stage of labour, she is fully dilated and ready to push. Pushing is a process that is inherent to all of us. We do it every time we have to have a bowel movement, the difference being that a baby is much larger and is coming out from an area that has never experienced this sensation. The act of pushing can be done in many positions, but if the woman is unable to assume these various positions, pushing may be slightly limited.

Pushing

As I mentioned before, my analogy of the key and lock really holds true as we need to continuously reassess the woman while she is pushing to determine if the head is engaged at the right angle within the pelvis. Certain positions will facilitate the descent of the head into the pelvis a lot easier and a lot faster. So I often tell women to keep an open mind in terms of which position they can adopt to push.

Mothers can use gravity to facilitate this by using a birthing chair, or they can squat. In a situation where the head is in the OP (occipital posterior) position the best way to bring the head around into the occipital anterior position, which is the preferable position for delivering the baby, is to get the woman on her hands and knees to push.

I believe that it is often difficult to try and get the woman to understand these positions ahead of time. That's the job of the person delivering you, so that they can better facilitate the delivery. It would be like a mover teaching you how to maneuver a desk through a door at the various angles he has learnt while he is still moving your furniture.

In any case, once you have pushed for a set period of time, the head should start to come down until finally there is an increased pressure as if you are going to have a bowel movement. There is also an increased sense of burning in the perineal area, which again is consistent with the baby's head coming down.

Once the head presents itself at the introitus or perineal area, there is a burning sensation called the 'ring of fire'. This is when you tend to hold back and not want to push any further! It's as if you are standing at the open door of an airplane ready to jump out with your parachute, but each time you step up to the open door you hold back, because you are just not ready to do it. This is often the case at this stage of pushing, where the woman just does not like that burning sensation. I often encourage her to push through this burning ring of fire, and this is what will enable the baby's head to go beyond the perineum and be delivered.

If the woman is allowed to stretch slowly at these final stages, once the head delivers, the perineum remains intact, and if there is a slight tear, this can be repaired a lot more easily and with fewer problems in the future.

It is at these final stages that the full cooperation of the mother is required. Once the head is pushed to a certain point, there is often a reflex from the mother to push the head further; once you parachute out of this plane, there is no coming back.

I often stress my point in the birthing plan that if there is anything that a woman should remember, it is not to push but to pant. My record to date is delivering an 11 lb 5 oz baby without a tear. This did take cooperation with the woman panting through each contraction, as the head was slowly delivered. I have often also used a coughing technique whereby I get the woman to cough in between contractions, which again facilitates the baby's head and avoids tearing.

An episiotomy *should* be performed if there is fetal distress in the presence of the crowning of the fetus's head, where the head needs to be delivered immediately. It is often performed in conjunction with a forceps delivery. Once the baby's head is delivered, I will suction the baby and then proceed to deliver the baby's shoulders and body.

I often hear from women that their first delivery was horrible because the baby almost died. In listening further to the story, it turns out that all that has really happened is that the baby was delivered and taken to the side table and suctioned and given a little bit of oxygen. This was interpreted as a near-death experience for the baby. It is crucial for parents to appreciate that one out of two babies are not given immediately to the mother, purely because the baby is reasonably flat on delivery. If the baby is delivered with vigorous crying and movement, generally the baby is given to the mother, the cord is clamped and cut, and there is no rush to do anything further at that point. But if the baby is reasonably flat, then the recommendation is to take the baby to the side table under a heated area with dry towels to stimulate the baby. This is generally all that is needed.

Once weighed and assessed, the baby is given back to the mother and any stitching that is required occurs at this point.

The third stage of labour is the delivery of the placenta. Potential problems arise in its delivery, as well as possible bleeding before or after its delivery. Excessive blood loss is called a postpartum hemorrhage and should be addressed by means of oxytoxics, which contract the uterus down so that there is no further blood loss.

Other Options

Well, we have pretty much gone through the easy part. Now we get to the stuff you really don't want to hear. For example, let's suppose that you were to dilate to 5 cm, that you do not progress in spite of good contractions, and then your uterus started to tire out. One of our options is an augmentation of labour, which can be done at any time once your labour has begun. In other words, we increase your uterine contractions if they are not adequate enough or not frequent enough. This is done intravenously and is similar to the oxytoxics we give once the placenta has been delivered, but it is given in smaller quantities and titrated up according to the frequency duration and intensity of the contractions.

We consider this failure to progress beyond the four hours. The rule of thumb is that in a first-timer (also known as a primip), the cervix should dilate at about 1 cm an hour, and in a multip (one or more delivered babies) at about 1.5 cm an hour, but this is quite a difficult rule of thumb to hold true. We certainly don't accept that in active labour the mother should take more than four hours to progress without some form of timeline of intervention.

Once a patient is fully dilated and has pushed without the baby descending, or if the baby is descending but becomes distressed, the doctor can assist the delivery of the baby by means of forceps or vacuum. This is only attempted if the head is low enough. Because of the complications arising in previous years from forceps deliveries, in North America, a forceps delivery can only be performed by an obstetrician. Forceps blades resembling salad tongs are applied to the baby's head, which is then either rotated or directly brought down. This is done without force and without any compromise to the baby. This is a much better route to go than to undergo a C-section.

Quite often women are frustrated because they have pushed for two hours, then a forceps attempt was made, and they ended up having a C-section anyway. We do this because we need to allow a full trial of labour to occur. If we don't give it our best shot, we can't know how simple and uncomplicated this labour and delivery might turn out to be. Many times I have seen a woman push for two hours and still have to have a C-section. This would be quite well predetermined if the head just did not progress during the course of those two hours. In my opinion, even though the guidelines call for the mother to push for two hours, I believe there are certainly exceptions where one can see that this is not working. This condition is called cephalopelvic disproportion (CPD) or obstructed labour.

Often parents worry about what a vacuum will do to the baby's head, making it into a cone head. This is a very short lived situation and the cone head is usually gone within 24 hours. Sometimes a bruise may occur, called a cephalhematoma. Although this may take several months to be reabsorbed, it does not result in any long-term problems.

Episiotomy

Women often worry about an episiotomy. This is an extremely old-fashioned procedure, involving cutting the perineal tissue to make extra room for the baby's head to avoid tearing into the rectal area. However, it is extremely rare for a natural tear to occur into the rectum, and over time doctors have recognized that an episiotomy is unnecessary.

An episiotomy *is* performed in an acute life-threatening situation where the baby needs to come out right away and where facilitation at the perineal level is essential. An episiotomy is also commonly performed when something like a forceps delivery is necessary. There are times however when the mother never progresses to the point of pushing while in the first stage of labour. The fetal monitor tells us if the baby is in acute distress, and if an emergency C-section is called for.

Cesarean Section

A Cesarean section (C-section) is the medical term for the surgical delivery of a baby from a woman's uterus. The incidence of C-section deliveries varies greatly according to the medical centre, and often the country, and can be seen as a measure of the quality of obstetrics in that particular community. In Canada, about 25.6 percent of women have C-section births.

In some cases, C-sections are planned for in advance, either because there is a contra-indication to vaginal birth or because a previous delivery resulted in a C-section, and there was an absolute reason for it being repeated.

Many C-sections occur as an emergency while the patient is in labour and because the labour is prolonged without advancing. That is, the labour fails to progress, and in spite of good strong contractions, the cervix stops its dilatation, or the baby fails to descend within the pelvis in spite of good effective pushing. A C-section also sometimes occurs in spite of attempts to deliver the baby vaginally by means of forceps or vacuum. And if at any point during labour the baby shows signs of significant distress, a C-section may also become necessary.

The baby's wellbeing is usually initially observed with external fetal monitoring. An external Doppler monitor picks up the fetal heart rate, which is correlated to the contractions of the mother. The monitor can be interpreted by your doctor or midwife. Sometimes there can be an indication that the baby is tiring or that the baby has developed a compromise to its blood flow from the placenta. If there is a concern, an internal fetal monitor can be used, which is a clip placed on the head of the fetus to detect a more accurate heart recording. If the fetal distress is worsening or showing certain patterns, then the doctor may need to intervene with a more active role such as an assisted vaginal delivery or with an emergency C-section.

The pendulum tends to swing back and forth in terms of the topic of VBAC, which stands for Vaginal Birth After C-section. C-sections used to be performed in such a way that the uterus was cut vertically, also called an up-down incision. This incision resulted in an inherent weakness in the uterine muscle with future pregnancies and resulted in the saying, "once a C-section, always a C-section". The incision is now rarely made today and has been replaced by a horizontal cut of the lower segment of the uterus. This has resulted in more women trying a VBAC delivery. A recent paper showed that in spite of this newer incision, there was a 1 percent incidence of fetal demise from acute uterine rupture during labour. This statistic has again made VBAC a judgment call. So I usually discuss the statistics with women deciding on whether to have a VBAC delivery or not. Some will immediately opt for an elective C-section.

I use a practical approach, so we look at why the initial C-section occurred. There are many cases where there is no doubt that the woman had a fair trial of labour and in spite of all the correct parameters, still went on to have a C-section. These women have often had a normal-sized baby who was correctly positioned, and in the big picture they are very unlikely to succeed with VBAC.

Then there is the woman who truly had very little trial of labour and would be ideal for a VBAC. A good example would be a woman who had a breech (bottom first) baby resulting in a C-section and now has a second normal vertex (head down) baby.

Placenta

The delivery of the placenta is considered the last part of labour and is referred to as the third stage of labour. The delivery of the placenta is crucial in order for the uterus to completely contract down and to end the final chapter we call labour.

There are complications seen at this stage. Sometimes the placenta can fail to separate from the uterus and result in a retained placenta. This is often associated with a lengthy waiting process. An hour of trying unsuccessfully to remove the placenta by means of a traction technique that is intermittently applied to the umbilical cord will result in a need to manually remove the placenta. This is easy to do in experienced hands, but needs some form of regional anesthesia or a general anesthetic in order to relax the pelvic muscles and also in order to minimize any further pain.

Once the placenta is out, it is inspected to ensure that there are three blood vessels (two arteries and one vein), and that there is no portion missing, which would mean that the uterus would be unable to contract fully, and that the woman might then bleed more, resulting in a postpartum hemorrhage or PPH. This usually requires a scraping procedure called a D & C done under anesthetic to remove this small, retained portion of the placenta.

Sometimes the uterus can bleed after the placenta is delivered because the uterine muscle has a poor tone. This is more common in women who have had more than one pregnancy, also referred to as multips. For this reason, oxytocin, a hormone that is naturally made in the pituitary gland, is released when the suckling newborn stimulates the nipple. Most medical professionals routinely inject this hormone in its synthetic form at the conclusion of labour.

After the Birth

Baby Stuff

Cord Blood

One very topical issue is the storage of your newborn's cord blood. Lifebank is a local company in British Columbia, Canada, that stores cord blood in liquid nitrogen, for an initial charge of about $1000 dollars and then an annual fee of $125 to store it until needed. There are many local such private banks throughout Canada and in the States.

The umbilical cord is rich in stem cells, which are the precursors to all cell-based organs in the human body. They can potentially be used in patients as a better option than bone-marrow transplant for patients with blood-borne cancers such as leukemia and Hodgkin's lymphoma and in sickle cell anemia.

Because stem cells can develop cells for any organ system, they are considered to be a possible future treatment for myriad of diseases, such as multiple sclerosis, lupus, Alzheimer's, Parkinson's, amyotrophic lateral sclerosis (ALS), diabetes, stroke, and diseases of the liver, kidneys, spinal cord, etc.

The advantage of using a bank at this point is a matter of contention. We are still many years away from using stem cells in such a diverse way. One view is that stem cells can be used on any individual, and that if use of them advances, this would result in private or government-run banks, which would not be money-driven and which would provide the donated cord blood to those in need. Several banks are currently being developed with a view to non-profit stem-cell provision.

Many people feel they can put their money to better use by establishing an educational fund using their cord-bank contributions over 18 years to equal a substantial return for their child's college education. I tend to agree with them.

Apgar Score

The Apgar score is a subjective assessment of the baby at birth, and at 1, 5, and 10 minutes following birth. Five things are assessed, each being scored out of 2, for a total possible score of 10.

Score	0	1	2
The heart rate	absent	below 100	above 100
Respiratory effort	absent	weak	good, strong cry
Muscle tone	limp	some flexion	active movement
Stimulus to the baby	no response	grimace	cry
Colour	blue/pale	pink body/extremities	all pink/ blue

A score of 7 to 10 is regarded as a good score. A score of 3 to 6 requires intervention with a mask and an airway in the mouth. Apgar of 0 to 2 indicates that acute resuscitation is required. A more objective way of assessing the fetus at birth is to exam the arterial and venous blood cord gases taken from the blood vessels of the placenta shortly after delivery. These give us a far more objective insight as to how the baby was at birth in terms of distress or fatigue. The blood gases take a while to process and also require a blood gas machine being available.

The newer neonatal resuscitation criteria do not advocate waiting 60 seconds for an Apgar score to determine if there is a need to intervene. The Apgar score is still recorded, but it is not useful for resuscitation purposes and it is not an accurate measure of how well the baby was at birth. It is more of a subjective measure.

Newborn Care

There truly is no manual with your new package, but the fundamental basics include keeping the baby warm, fed and nurtured.

All newborns enter into a due protocol when born in a hospital setting. They are treated with erythromycin antibiotic ointment applied in the first hour to both eyes. This reduces any potential eye infection. Parents often ask me not to do this, as they are concerned that it will affect the baby. The ointment does not sting or hurt the baby, and it does not cause any visual compromise in that the baby does not have normal vision in the first few weeks anyway. The ointment prevents any eye infection that might require future application of the same ointment 4 to 6 times a day for seven days.

Babies are fragile in the beginning and potentially have a tendency to bleed due to an insufficient clotting mechanism. For this reason vitamin K is injected into newborns within the first 6 hours of birth.

Certain diseases can be present in apparently healthy newborns and if untreated can cause irreversible mental retardation. Phenylketonuria hyperphenylalaninemia occurs in about 1 in 18,000 babies and is treated with a special diet. Congenital hypothyroidism occurs in 1 in 3,000 to 4,000 babies and is treated by giving the baby thyroid pills daily. Galactosemia occurs in 1 in 30,000 babies and is treated with a special diet. Medium Chain Acyl-CoA Dehydrogenase deficiency (MCAD) is seen in 1 in 12,000 babies and treated with diet. These four diseases are all tested for after 24 hours of birth.

Premature Babies

This term refers to babies born before 37 weeks. Because their organ systems are developed but immature, they do need extra care and usually end up in a special care unit.

Some of the problems resulting from premature births are:

♦ Immature lungs causing breathing problems. This may result in closer monitoring of the blood oxygen saturation levels and also some assistance with extra oxygen and sometimes with ventilation.

♦ Uncoordinated sucking and swallowing resulting in feeding difficulties.

♦ Increased chance of infection due to an immature immune system.

♦ Heat temperature regulation problems.

♦ Immature liver making jaundice more likely.

♦ More fragile blood vessels will result in higher chance of bruising and bleeding making it more important to handle gently.

This also is an extremely tough time for parents. I truly can understand what this does to a parent both professionally and personally. Our son Taylor was born with respiratory distress and was in a special care nursery with oxygen ventilation for 21 days. These were truly 21 days of hell. There is always frustration, anger, guilt and probably every emotion of loss that a parent can go through. All your expectations are crushed; you are emotionally drained. It is a time when you have to believe in medical expertise and to have a solid belief system. It is also a time when you need love and support from your family and friends.

Low Birth-Weight Babies

There is a direct correlation between length of pregnancy and birth weight. One third of low birth-weight babies, however, are born at term. Some factors that can affect a baby's birth weight include the sex of the baby, status and race of the parents, prenatal care including nutrition and weight, multiple births, and maternal factors such as alcohol or drug abuse and illness. These babies are often managed and treated exactly like premature babies because they have the same problems.

So, now the problems begin: you have this wonderful baby, you are in a hospital, and now you have issues, questions, concerns and anxieties. Guess what—they are only going to get worse, so you might as well enjoy this new chapter in your life. Here are some things, however, that you can consider that might help guide you and give you some reassurance.

Breastfeeding

You are about to breastfeed and have no clue what to do and you wonder what the best approach is. Well, truly this is a technique that you will learn just as your baby will. You are a new team. The most important thing that I can tell you is to try and start off correctly. You want your baby to breastfeed with the entire nipple and areola area in the baby's mouth, not just the tip of the nipple. The baby can thus 'latch' on rather than suction on. This will reduce the surface area upon which the baby suckles and therefore reduce the amount of discomfort and problems, such as cracked and sore nipples.

Initiating breastfeeding soon after delivery has many benefits. It starts an immediate bonding process. Probably, of even more significance, it causes the amino acid oxytocin to be released from the pituitary gland, and this causes the uterus to contract, resulting in less blood loss from the uterus. It is also this uterine stimulation that results in 'after pains'.

This amino acid (octapeptide) has also been synthesized based on the physiological properties of oxytocin and is applied clinically to induce (initiate) and augment (increase the intensity and frequency of) labour, and to stop bleeding after delivery. Oxytocin is routinely given after delivery, in most centres. Some doctors prefer to give it after the baby's anterior shoulder is delivered, and others may give it once the placenta has delivered. Over the years I have found that giving it after the placenta is delivered results in fewer retained placentas in my practice.

Remember that in the beginning it is impossible to know if your baby is getting enough breast milk and this is why weighing the baby is so vital. Each baby has a different schedule in the beginning. Some will cluster feed and others feed continuously with breaks in between. So some clues that the baby is getting enough are that he feeds at least 8 times a day, is satisfied after a feed, swallows well when feeding, has 5 to 6 wet cloth diapers a day or 4 to 5 disposable diapers after the third day of birth, and has soft stools 2 to 3 times a day in the first month. Another indication is that your breasts are full before feeds and soft after feeds.

Please bear in mind that I am not a lactation specialist, nor do I profess to be an expert on breastfeeding, but this is a process that may take a good 2 to 3 weeks to learn and to be accomplished in. As difficult as it sounds there is no better approach than good old, natural breastfeeding in the initial stages of your baby's life.

Remember that initially the only milk you produce is a very thin form called colostrum. It is very rich and gives your baby nutrition and protection against sickness. Start off breastfeeding by being comfortable and by making sure that your baby is comfortable too. Positioning is an essential part of this.

As I am sure you already know, the advantages are endless. They include bonding with your baby, providing the most natural form of nutrition, and passing on passive immunoglobulins, which will give your baby protection against most illnesses in the first three months. There is one last added bonus to breastfeeding—it burns 500 calories a day. It is a very effective way of losing weight!

To toughen up the areola area after each breastfeed, you can rub on some lanolin, or you can express some colostrum and use an ordinary 60-watt light bulb in a lamp to dry the colostrum on the areola and nipple area. It will take several days for your breast milk to come in, then the breasts become hard and engorged, and the baby can start to feed and gain weight.

Bottle Feeding

If you have decided not to breastfeed, you need to be prepared with bottles, bottle nipples, formula and boiling apparatus. There are many varieties of bottles out there. The best I have seen is an L-shaped bottle, such as the Playtex Advance, with an air escape valve that prevents the infant swallowing air. Like all plastic bottles, they need to be boiled in order to sterilize them. Check if your dishwasher has a sterilizing mode to save you boiling bottles.

A great variety of different-shaped teats are available to choose from. Often one is more suitable than another for your infant, and you may have to try a few types to find the one she prefers. The best orthodontically engineered nipple is the NUK® nipple and it is probably the best first choice. Check how fast the milk drips out of the nipple. Again this is another reason I like the L-shaped bottle because the air valve regulates the milk flow.

An easy feeding schedule to remember is:

0-3 weeks	8-10 feeds daily of 2-3 ounces/60-100ml
1-4 months	6-8 feeds daily of 4-5 ounces/125-150ml
4-6 months	4-6 feeds daily of 30-40 oz/900-1200ml
6-12 months	3-5 feeds daily of 24-32 oz/720- 960 ml

Formula

There are a vast number of formula products to choose from. Each formula has its own particular potential benefits. The bottom line is to find one your baby likes and that agrees with him so that he does not become colicky or fussy from intolerance to the formula. A good starting type is a regular formula that is milk-based, not a soy-based one or a lactose-free one. I usually start a formula-fed baby on Good Start®. "Good Start® seems to be so well tolerated because it is easy to digest. It is the only infant formula that is made with 100% whey protein that has been partially broken down. The partial breakdown results in its ease of being absorbed and processed. In addition it is the only routine starter formula clinically shown to reduce allergic symptoms in babies who have a family history of allergies." I seldom find the need in switching once initiating with this particular brand. If, however there are any difficulties I will switch to one of the others.

A very good formula I use for babies who regurgitate is Enfamil® A+ with rice starch. This has a unique ingredient that expands in the stomach and reduces regurgitation quite substantially.

Research has shown that breast milk has omega-3 and omega-6 fatty acids that are crucial for development of the brain in infants. Several formula companies have added these ingredients to their infant formulas, and advertise them as formula with docosahexaenoic acid or DHA (omega-3) and arachidonic acid or ARA (omega-6). Soy-based formulas are used for babies with sensitivity to cows milk protein, and lactose-free formulas are used for babies having trouble digesting lactose. As a clinician, I must admit that the distinction between the two is quite difficult.

All formulas have vitamins and iron so that formula-fed babies generally require no additional vitamin or iron supplements. Some formulas have extra iron, which may increase the consistency of the baby's stool and may also make a baby more colicky.

Specific formulas are available for 6 months and through to 18 months. These 'next step' formulas are supposed to have a benefit in being adapted as a next step for the more mature infant.

My preferred approach is to switch over from the initial formula once 12 months is reached. The toddler is now mature enough to tolerate cows milk.

Mix water with formula for the powders that need reconstitution, but remember that this water is to be boiled and cooled for infants up to 3 months of age.

Sometimes a baby can have a real hard time feeding from a bottle or breast because of a remnant of skin found under the tongue, called a frenulum. It is present in all of us, attached underneath the tongue at the back, but in some babies it extends to closer to the tip. These babies are quite literally tongue-tied. A minor procedure done by a pediatrician within a few days of birth cuts the frenulum to correct the tongue. There is also an upper frenulum attaching the upper gum to the part just above the upper front teeth. This does not cause a problem with feeding but as the upper front teeth develop, a gap forms between the teeth, forming the 'Madonna' or 'David Letterman' gap. This truly is a cosmetic issue but again can be dealt with at an early age to avoid this look.

Feeding Difficulties

One of the first crises I see is within the first week, where weight is lost, but not regained. Acceptable weight loss is up to 10% of the baby's initial birth weight. So for example if a baby weighs in at 3000 gm, we will accept 300 gm weight loss in the first week. Weight loss beyond 10% can lead to the large problem of the mother feeling guilty because she is having problems breastfeeding. The baby is having difficulty latching on; a lactation consultant is called in. So many other nurses are involved in the mother's initial care that she is bombarded with suggestions for different techniques and different approaches. And all consistently guilting her into feeling that she is compelled to breastfeed.

Breast nipple confusion is of great concern, and so a lactation consultant will often ensure that the only other substitute to breast-feeding is by a dropper or a sipping cup or both. My approach is a little bit less conservative. I have yet to see a confused baby when it comes to breastfeeding versus bottle-feeding. My approach is very simple. If the baby is failing to thrive and the mother is unable to produce enough milk, or the baby is unable to latch on to facilitate enough colostrum and breast milk in the first week, I have adopted something which I refer to as the 10-10-10 rule. This allows the mother an alternative to both pumping and breastfeeding and essentially exhausting herself in that first week. This exhaustion often sets her up for instant failure. The 10-10-10 rule is simple in that the baby will feed 10 minutes on one breast, 10 minutes on the other breast and will be topped up with 10 minutes on a bottle with formula. This is hardly harmful for the baby and, as I have said, I have never seen any confusion occur.

This ensures that the baby does gain weight and also allows the mother enough sleep time that her breast milk will come in. She will then be able to increase the amount of time the baby is on each breast and reduce the amount of time of the bottle feed over the course of one to two weeks.

Breast/Nipple Confusion

This is often a big concern for parents who are told to never confuse their baby by offering a bottle over the breast. The idea is that once the baby is exposed to that evil bottle, she is going to get confused and turn to the bottle.

I have yet to see this type of confusion. Now, don't get me wrong: breast is best. But I have faith in the natural instinct of a baby to recognize mom by the smell of her breast milk. That same baby is going to choose the easier mode of the two and that is most often the breast. A baby turns to a bottle when the breast mode is not working, and this is usually a cue to switch over at this point. There are already far too many moms who are made to feel guilty over a hopeless situation, and the guilt should not be prolonged.

Weight Gain

In the first week I expect a weight loss in a breast-fed baby. If a baby is bottle-fed there is usually very little weight loss. My general rule is that once a baby has had an initial loss of weight up to 10%, I expect a weight gain of around one ounce per day. If the gain is less than that, I look for reasons. The most common one is that the mom is not producing enough milk. A drug called Motilium®, or domperidone, can be given to increase milk production, and in the interim, the mom can pump with a rental electrical unit. Hand pumps are usually inadequate and are a waste of money. The 10-10-10 rule is a practical alternative, but I will sometimes have moms who are really opposed to any formula and are willing to endure the latter option of breast and pumping.

Supplements

Newborn babies should be supplemented with vitamin D, especially here in Canada where we tend to have reasonably short summers and where sun exposure is at a minimum. The exception to supplementing is for babies whose formula is already enriched with vitamin D and other vitamins.

Fluoride is a controversial supplement. All dentists agree that in those provinces or states with fluoridation of the municipal water supply, the incidence of dental caries and tooth decay are remarkably less. As a result, many dentists have advocated in the past that all infants should be given fluoride drops as early as one month of age in areas without water fluoride treatment. This is somewhat confusing, as most doctors do not recommend supplementing with fluoride until the eruption of the first tooth. And to further confuse things, there are many proponents against fluoridation of water supplies. Too much fluoride causes toxicity in children that causes teeth to crumble and makes bones brittle.

So, as a loving parent, what do *you* do as far as fluoride supplements go? If your water supply has fluoridation, no supplements are needed. If you do not have fluoride in your water supply, be more aware of the chances of dental caries but do not supplement with oral fluoride. For teeth and their care, refer to that section of this book.

Solids

The old guidelines recommended that babies be fed by breast or bottle until 4 months. At four months, you could start adding rice cereal. Once tolerated, vegetables and fruits could be added starting at one-week intervals. This method of introduction of a new fruit or vegetable would identify anything your child might be sensitive to. Once you reached the six-month mark, you could slowly introduce poultry and meat, and milk products.

Things to avoid up until one year were unpasteurized products, especially unpasteurized honey, as well as shellfish and egg white.

The new guidelines advocate that solids should only be started after 6 months, especially if there is a strong family history of allergies, as this reduces the risk of developing allergies.

My approach is to go with the new guidelines unless a baby shows a drop in weight at the 4-month visit relative to his or her percentile. In addition, if the baby is now waking up hungry, this is an indication that he needs more calories to sustain him on his percentile, and that milk alone is not capable of doing it. Given this scenario, I usually will introduce solids, unless this child has a strong family history of allergies.

Bowel Movements

Some parents worry because their baby has pooped 10 times in one day; some parents worry because he only pooped once in 10 days. The biggest issue for me is not the frequency, but the consistency. Is it hard like pebbles, or is it nice and soft and mushy? How distressed is the baby?

Colour and consistency will change according to the breast milk, the foods that mom ingests, and also if the baby is receiving formula. The colour of the stool usually tells me nothing. If we have a reasonably happy baby and the stool is nice and soft, then I have no concerns. Newborns have very loose and runny stools. If they are being bottle-fed, correct preparation is important. Bottles and nipples need to be sterilized by boiling during the first three months. The water for mixing formula powder is to be boiled and cooled before use. Always prepare bottles with well-washed hands. I will always remember the admission of one of my newborns after a severe bout of diarrhea due to salmonella passed on from chicken preparation.

Diarrhea and Vomiting

A virus, or bacteria or something even more obvious such as eating unusual kinds or amounts of food can cause diarrhea or vomiting. An infant is sometimes unable to tolerate large amounts of juice, fruit, or even milk. Breast-fed babies are less likely to develop diarrhea. Stomach flu often starts with vomiting, sometimes followed in a few hours by diarrhea, sometimes without diarrhea.

Infants and children under ages 4, and especially younger than 6 months, can dehydrate easily and need special attention when they have diarrhea or are vomiting. If the baby is newborn to 2 years and is breast-fed, continue to breast-feed. If the diarrhea is getting worse or the child is vomiting, then consider supplementing with a children's oral electrolyte. If the baby is formula-fed, switch to an oral electrolyte solution and gradually add back formula feeding within 24 hours. Do *not* use sports drinks to treat dehydration as they contain too much sugar and not enough minerals. For children over 2 years, you can use diluted Gatorade or another sports drinks if the diarrhea is mild to moderate.

The most common cause of serious viral gastroenteritis resulting in dehydration and hospitalization is the rotavirus, which occurs every year seasonally in Canada between November and June. This extremely challenging virus is highly resilient; as a result, conventional forms of prevention such as hand washing, antiseptics and disinfectants fail to prevent its spread. It is therefore very contagious. It is commonly associated with fever, vomiting, and diarrhea of up to 20 watery stools in one day. This is why dehydration is so common, with an annual worldwide death rate of 440,000 people.

Diaper Rash

This is a red rash seen over the babies' buttocks, perineum, or thigh area. It is usually uncomfortable but not serious and is caused by moisture and bacteria in a baby's urine and stools or as a reaction to soap used to wash cloth diapers or to products within disposable diapers.

I often find parents unknowingly mismanage diaper rashes. Prevention is obviously the key. This means changing diapers as soon as they are soiled and wet. If you are using cloth diapers, wash them in mild detergent soaps like Ivory Snow, and double rinse. ***Do not use bleach.*** After a diaper change, dry the bottom well, so that it is completely dry and if you are going to apply a barrier, use Vaseline®.

Acidic stool may also be causing the rash. If it is accompanied by frothy diarrhea, I will use oral Ovol® to reduce the acidity, in addition to taking the precautions above.

If you are still battling, consider a different brand of disposable diapers. If your choice is cloth diapers, avoid plastic pants.

The general tendency is to reach for the zinc-based, barrier creams, which I find do not always help with this situation. I believe diaper rash occurs for several reasons, but once the skin is sensitized, it often gets worse when a zinc-based cream retains some of the moisture between the layer of the zinc and the skin. This results in a yeast fungal infection.

For this reason I recommend Vaseline ointment, or failing this, one of the combination ointments, such as an antifungal ointment with a mild corticosteroid. Failing this, I often incorporate an anti-burn cream called Flamazine®, and this sometimes can be extremely beneficial.

Urinary Crystals

These often appear within the first few days of birth. They look like blood in the diaper and are the result of precipitation of concentrated uric acid crystals due to an initial dehydration in the newborn baby. Although they are of concern to parents, they disappear within the first week.

Circumcision

I try to use a common sense approach in advising parents when it comes to circumcision, which is the surgical removal of the foreskin. There is no data to support the theory that circumcision has any benefits, and it is performed for personal and/or religious reasons. I have very rarely seen complications, the most common problem being some adhesions of the remnant foreskin sticking to the head of the penis. This is easily treated with a corticosteroid topical cream. Depending on the technique used, the amount of pain is negligible. I usually see more problems in kids who are not circumcised and now require a procedure under general anesthetic. (This statistic is as high as 6%.) Problems often result from a very tight foreskin, which may result in recurrent infection in the head and foreskin of the penis. I often recommend that circumcised fathers have their boys circumcised their boys, as they have less experience they can pass on in foreskin maintenance.

The techniques done vary according to the doctor. Mogen circumcision seems to be very successful in one of the circumcision clinics in Vancouver and has been used by religious rabbis for hundreds of years. It takes 40 seconds, and is often accompanied by topical and then an injected freezing. Parents have often come back to me amazed that their infant slept right through the procedure.

Of the two other methods, the Gomco Clamp is a more traditional method and takes longer. The Plastibell is a plastic device that is tied to the penis. The foreskin dies over several days.

Nipples and Breasts

The nipples of infants may be hard and the size of a peanut, due to the breast buds found in all newborns regardless of sex. Estrogen from breast milk, and sometimes, in formula-fed babies, directly from the mother during pregnancy affects an infant's breast buds making them hard.

Cord

The cord is clamped at birth with a cord clamp. The stump dries out and a health professional then removes the clamp with a special clamp remover. In the past, the cord was cleaned on a regular basis with alcohol, but this actually delayed separation of the cord at its base from the baby's belly button. The cord is now left alone. It undergoes a natural process during which it starts to smell, and a purulent and bloody-type discharge often occurs before the cord finally falls off. Parents who are concerned about the discharge usually bring their newborn in at about day 5. The discharge rarely poses a problem, but is usually a sign that the cord will fall off soon. Once the cord is off, I always apply some hydrogen peroxide on a Q-tip to the area. It fizzes and bubbles nicely, cleaning the entire area of the remaining smelly pus.

Occasionally there is a defect in the area called an umbilical hernia; this will usually disappear gradually. If it is not gone after one year, it may need surgical repair, but this is rare.

Newborn Skin

Peeling skin is common in newborns, especially in a baby born beyond its due date. The solution is a good over-the-counter hydrating, moisturizing cream. A waxy substance that looks like butter or lard, known as vernix, may cover the body of babies who are premature or preterm. Surprisingly though, we also sometimes see this in babies who are term or postdates.

Baby Acne and Skin problems

Baby acne usually occurs at one month of age. There is really nothing we can do, as the sweat glands start to produce sebum, which comes to the surface. The baby's glands are still immature and may not yet be capable of secreting the sebum, hence the appearance of baby acne. This is transient and disappears within a month.

Cradle cap (seborrheic dermatitis) is related to the thickness of the sebum that is produced in the scalp area and results in a thick yellowish plaque over the scalp. This is easily dealt with baby oil and can be brushed out of the baby's hair on a daily basis.

Sensitive dermatitis-type skin is fairly common in newborns. I often have moms coming in with the diagnosis of eczema and the first knee-jerk reaction is to give these little babies a cortisone-based cream. However, cortisone creams can cause depigmentation and thinning of the skin, so I tend to use these only if the inflammation is severe and requires acute intervention.

I prefer to look into the underlying cause, and we often find that it is a result of the choice of detergent. A baby-type detergent, such as Ivory Snow, is commonly a quick solution.

Sensitive skin is easily managed with precautions in bath products by using glycerin soap such as Neutrogena® glycerin soap on the skin and scalp. One to two tablespoons of baking soda in the bath will make the water soft and smooth like silk. An excellent cream for total body use is Cetaphil® Therapeutic Barrier Cream.

Teeth

At least once a day I am asked, "When will my baby get his teeth? 'Cause the books say…" The truth is that all babies are born with a full set of teeth. They are just covered by the gums. So it does not matter what the sequential set of events are meant to be. All babies eventually get their teeth and all of these teeth will eventually be replaced by permanent teeth. I have seen newborns with teeth and I have seen 12-monthers without any.

Teething will usually start with drooling, fussiness and sometimes fever. If the fever is high, always suspect that there is another cause. Treatment can be local with cold cloths or chewable teething rings, local topicals such as Orajel®, and—probably the most beneficial—Advil or Motrin which as anti-inflammatories will reduce the swelling in addition to the analgesic benefits.

Teeth should be brushed once they are poking through and should also be flossed regularly. Bottle-feeding before bed is a major cause of dental caries. If you feed before bed, brush before bed. Bottle-feeding should be stopped at 18 months or sooner to avoid caries.

Fluoride is an effective and inexpensive way to prevent tooth decay. Many communities automatically fluoridate their water systems. Fluoride supplements are supposed to be implemented at 3 years, but this is controversial as often tooth rot is seen a lot earlier.

Your baby's teeth will benefit by placing a smear of fluoride toothpaste on a clean wet cloth or baby toothbrush and wipe or brush every day. As your child gets older, increase the amount to a pea-sized amount on a baby toothbrush. Dental check-ups should begin at about 2 years old.

Soother or Thumb?

I think soothers are great. The alternative is a thumb, and thumb suckers are a huge medical challenge. The beauty about soothers is they can be removed—thumbs are not that readily removable and herein lies the challenge.

In addition, soother babies have a lower incidence of SIDS. Remember, however, that soothers should never be used as a substitute in a hungry child. Wait until breastfeeding has been established to introduce a soother, and implement correct dental hygiene to avoid the tooth decay that can accompany use of the soother.

Your goal should be to eliminate the soother when your child is about 12 months old.

Colic

Colic is a new mom's worst nightmare, as colicky babies are extremely fussy and difficult to please. It's not a disease, but is caused by abdominal pain believed to be due to intestinal gas.

All babies cry, so how do you confirm that your baby has colic? Colic usually follows the *rule of three*: crying starts within the first three months after birth and continues more than three hours a day, more than three days a week. As the baby and his bowels mature, colic goes away, usually by the third month from its onset. There are several things that can be looked at to try and rectify a colicky baby. First of all, how is she feeding? If she sounds as if she is choking with breastfeeding or bottle-feeding, it could be that she is sucking air in while feeding. For bottles, changing the nipple or the aperture of the teat could rectify this. Air can be sucked in if the nipple hole is too small or too big. A good rule of thumb is to assess the flow by using cold formula and checking that it flows at about one drop per second. Make sure that you are not overheating the formula; it should be at body temperature.

A mom who is breastfeeding can express some of the milk before feeding, so that the velocity and volume at which the milk comes out of the breast is altered.

Babies need to suck on something for up to two hours a day to be satisfied. If feedings are not enough, use a pacifier.

You can also try to reduce the amount of gas with products such as Ovol drops, gripe water, or fennel tea. Fennel is a herb that smells similar to licorice. It is traditionally used in drugs to treat stomach problems. Buy it at health food stores, and make it into tea. You can drink it hot, or you could also cool it down and drop it into your baby's mouth just as you would Ovol and gripe water.

When your baby is in colic mode, try to distract her, by rocking or walking her, placing her in the football position, so that she is placed on your forearm stomach down. A car ride or outdoor stroll, or an external noise such as a clothes dryer or vacuum or a bubbling aquarium, or television or music can all be worth trying.

Jaundice

Jaundice is one of the most frequent things that I see in a newborn. Typically it becomes apparent about 2 to 4 days after birth.

About half of full term and two thirds of premature newborns get some degree of jaundice, called physiological jaundice, in which the eyes and skin of the baby take on a yellow tinge. The newborn is breaking down blood in the body that worked when they were in utero, but is no longer needed. The broken-down blood becomes bilirubin, which is removed by the liver. The bilirubin can only be processed at a certain rate, and if the liver is not able to cope, the bilirubin accumulates in the blood, resulting in the yellow tinge of jaundice. If a baby becomes very yellow, or is very lethargic, this could indicate high levels of bilirubin. Appropriate levels of bilirubin depend upon the baby's age and size, and on whether the baby is term or pre-term.

Bilirubin is measurable in the blood, and if it remains above a certain level phototherapy can be initiated. The treatment is done in hospital by placing the baby under special UV lights. Alternatively, increasing the frequency of feeds and placing the baby in a room with indirect sun exposure will often solve the problem.

Two other forms of infant jaundice are recognized. Jaundice that occurs within 24 hrs of birth is usually considered to be pathological. It is due to uncommon causes such as hemolysis (destruction of blood) and sepsis (a condition or syndrome caused by the presence of bacteria in the blood circulation). Jaundice that occurs between days 4 to 7 in breastfed babies is called breast-milk jaundice and can last from 3 to 12 weeks. Its causes are still under investigation, but it is thought to be caused by a substance inside the breast milk that inhibits an enzyme called uridine diphospho-glucuronic acid (UDPGA) glucuronyl transferase, resulting in an accumulation of unconjugated bilirubin pigment in the skin.

Physiologic jaundice results from the immaturity of the newborn's liver and its inability to produce enough UDPGA glucuronyl transferase, which is required to conjugate bilirubin. Conjugated bilirubin is water-soluble and can be excreted, but the unconjugated form cannot be excreted, so it builds up in the blood and is then deposited into the skin.

Some research shows that lipoprotein lipase, found in some breast milk, produces nonesterified long-chain fatty acids, which competitively inhibit glucuronyl transferase conjugating activity. This activity is needed to convert bilirubin from its unconjugated form to its conjugated form in the liver. Glucuronidase has also been found in some breast milk, which results in jaundice. The treatment of this problem is to stop breastfeeding and to switch to formula. On a more practical level, I find it easier to do several things. You can pump for one to two weeks and in the interim exclusively formula feed until the jaundice resolves. Another option is to alternate days with formula one day and breast milk the next. A last option is to alternate feeds each day from breast to formula. This should not be a substitute for phototherapy intervention. The former options are usually applied in the more severe jaundice and the latter options in the less severe jaundice.

The only definitive measure of severity of jaundice is to measure bilirubin levels by doing a blood test. Kramer classified jaundice in its severity by looking at which parts of the baby were jaundiced. He noted that it started on the head and moved down, and this formed the basis of his classifications. In Zone 1—which is anywhere in the head region—jaundice is in its mildest form. Zone 2 extends into the trunk, Zone 3 into the abdomen and thighs, Zone 4 into the arms and shin/calf area, and finally Zone 5 extends to the feet and hands. If jaundice extends to Zone 5, this is obviously more serious than the other zones.

Thrush

Thrush is a yeast infection found in a newborn's mouth, but it can occur at any time until about 18 months. It causes a white cottage cheesy-looking plaque to grow inside the mouth, on the tongue, and on the cheeks. It is more common in the first 3 months, because a newborn has very few bacteria in his mouth. After 3 months, bacteria will start to develop in the mouth, causing the breath to smell. But once these 'good' bacteria start to thrive, they prevent yeast from growing in the mouth. Sometimes a baby can have a white furry tongue from milk, but this is not a yeast infection.

Most yeast infections are easy to treat with an anti-fungal drop such as Nilstat®. Some thrush infections are a challenge, however, and you will need to paint on Gentian violet. This is a very messy purple preparation; be careful not to spill it as it stains.

Strabismus

Strabismus is a congenital weakness of one of the muscles of the eye; it is often corrected by 4 months of age. If it does not, take your baby to a specialist. Sometimes the eyes appear to be out of alignment because of a flap of skin in both corners of the eyes, creating the illusion of strabismus. In babies with true strabismus, correct the eyes at an early stage to avoid problems of double vision.

Colds, Eye Infections and Tear ducts in Newborns

Many newborns have very small tear ducts and thus have a sluggish drainage from the eyes resulting in a tearing of the eyes. You can fix this quite easily with regular manual massage. Gently massage the inner corner of the eye, which is where the tear duct is located, and this usually allows better drainage of the eye. First, locate your own tear duct by placing your pinky finger at the inside corner of the eye where the upper and lower lids join. At this angle you can feel a small bump, which is the opening to the tear duct. Now you know where to find it, you can massage your baby's tear duct regularly, for example, each time the baby feeds.

In the case of an infected eye with pus and discharge I prescribe erythromycin ophthalmic ointment. This does not burn the eye and is the same ointment initially applied to a newborn in the delivery room. In older children I use an antibiotic eye drop called Vigamox™ that is very effective and is only needed 2 to 3 times a day.

New moms are often concerned that their newborn has developed a cold when they are in fact hearing nasal congestion, which is common. It can be due to one of two things. The first is the initial irritation of amniotic fluid on the nasal tissue at birth. Alternately, a significant amount of regurgitation occurs from the stomach. When newborns drink breast milk, it often regurgitates up into the back of the throat and into the nose. I rarely use an aspirator for this because I believe that it causes trauma to the nasal mucous membranes. I use a saline nose drop, which is salt water and the same consistency as natural tears. This flushes mucous from the nose down into the back of the throat.

Babies often throw up or spit up. If the baby is having a substantial feed, there will be a fair bit of reflux, because the baby's stomach is relatively small. A newborn has a poor valve mechanism between the stomach and the esophagus. This throw-up often looks much worse than it really is. The only time we really get concerned is when the baby is losing weight and when the throw-up becomes progressively worse.

Fontanelles and Sutures

Sutures are the dense connective tissues between the flat bones of the skull. They are fibrous joints that allow the skull to mould at the time of labour and permit the skull rapid enlargement with rapid growth of the brain up until five years of age, at which time both skull and brain are about the size of those of an average adult. Once fully grown, the flat bones fuse to become a solid skull.

There are six large fibrous areas called fontanelles. The most obvious and easily felt are the anterior (diamond-shaped) and posterior (triangular) fontanelles. As a rule, but not always, the posterior fontanelle closes within 2 to 3 months after birth as the surrounding bones grow. The anterior fontanelle closes by the 18th month. The two halves of the frontal bone normally begin to fuse during the 2nd year, and the frontal suture is often obliterated by the 8th year. The other sutures disappear during adult life, but the closing of sutures and fontanelles are often subject to wide variations.

A fontanelle in a clinical setting can sometimes provide additional information as to whether a baby is dehydrated or has increased pressure in the brain. This is the type of assessment that should only be interpreted by a clinician. Caregivers often ask me if a child is dehydrated because of this issue. I am usually able to reassure them. My sense is that this is something that parents need not worry about.

Purple Extremities

Often a baby will have blue or purple extremities, which will arouse concern about the infant's circulation in parents and friends. Unless your baby also has blue lips, face or tongue, you don't need to worry. Most infants have poor blood flow to their hands and feet, so that they are often blue.

Fever

What is fever? Fever is when the body's temperature rises above its normal level of around 37.0°C (98.6°F). The body's normal temperature does fluctuate throughout the day between 36.1°C (97°F) to 37.4°C (99.3°F), being lower in the morning and higher in the evening.

A temperature greater than 38°C (100.4°F) measured rectally, greater than 37.8°C (100.0°F) measured orally or in the ear, and greater than 37.2°C (99.9°F) measured under the arm are all values that are considered above normal.

One of our natural defenses against infection or illness is an elevated temperature, so a fever indicates that an infection or illness is present. It is important, therefore, to determine the cause of the fever. In children, viral infections, such as colds, flu, chickenpox, can cause fevers. Body temperature can also rise when an infant is overdressed or when a room is too warm.

There is no medical evidence that fevers from infection can cause brain damage. The body limits a fever caused by infection from going above 40.6 degrees Celsius (105 Fahrenheit). Heat from an external source (like sunshine on a parked car), however, can cause the body temperature to go above 41.1 (106F), and brain damage can then occur rapidly.

General management of fever is to encourage the child to drink extra fluids, the colder the better. Frozen popsicles or crushed ice slurpees are a fast method of lowering fever. Dress your child lightly and do not wrap her to sweat it out. If the fever is higher than 38.3 degrees (101 degrees F) and she is comfortable, give her acetaminophen or ibuprofen.

Febrile Convulsions

These are uncontrolled muscle spasms that can happen while a child's temperature is rapidly rising. Sometimes this can be the first sign that in fact she has a fever. Once her fever has reached a high temperature, the risk of a convulsion is probably over.

A child with a febrile convulsion will lose consciousness. The muscles will stiffen and the teeth will clench. Then the arms and legs start to jerk. The eyes may roll back, and she may stop breathing for a few seconds. She may vomit, urinate, or pass stools.

A convulsion may last 1 to 5 minutes, and although frightening for everyone, they are seldom serious. The most susceptible age is 6 months to 4 years. Of this age group, 2% to 4% are at risk of febrile convulsions.

To manage a convulsion while it is happening, is first of all, to stay calm. Protect your child from injury and position her on her side so that any saliva or vomit will clear her mouth and not obstruct her airways. Never put anything in her mouth to prevent tongue biting.

Following the convulsion, drowsiness is common, but your first priority is to lower the fever.

Congenital Hip Dislocation

The hip is a ball and socket joint that normally allows for a wide range of motion, while holding the leg securely in the joint. In some children, the joint is too lax, leading to instability of the hips. Although this is commonly called congenital hip dislocation, the hips are rarely dislocated at birth. The hips haven't developed completely, but the dislocation happens later on. The condition is more accurately called dislocatable hips or developmental dislocation of the hips (DDH).

Anyone can be born with DDH, but it tends to occur in families with a history of DDH, and is especially common in firstborn children. Hip instability is far more common in girls than in boys, and among those who are born in the breech position. It is often associated with congenital torticollis (a twisting or tilting of the neck due to a shortened neck muscle). If your baby has torticollis or turned in feet, pay careful attention to the hips.

You may notice that your baby has an unequal number of thigh skin folds, uneven knee position, or legs that appear to be different lengths. Most often, however, the instability is only noticed when a doctor feels a clunk when maneuvering the hips in a particular way during well-baby exams. The diagnosis is suspected on physical exam and confirmed with imaging studies. Hip clicks may be of concern to parents, but these usually do not represent a problem by themselves.

Ultrasound exam at 6 weeks is helpful in diagnosis. Until that time, a conservative treatment that is often effective in treating is double diapering. Parents put two diapers on their infant with each diaper change; this keeps the hips in a good position for this problem. Unless the problem is corrected before the baby begins to bear weight, long-term hip damage can occur. Treatment depends on the developmental status of the hips, and often involves holding the hips in the correct position to continue development. This might be accomplished with harnesses, splints, or other devices. Sometimes surgery is needed to correct the problem.

Often hip instability cannot be prevented. Avoiding excess exposure to estrogens or medicines that relax the hips, and avoiding breech delivery may prevent some cases.

Clubfoot

Clubfoot is a deformity of the foot and lower calf. The bones, joints, muscles, and blood vessels of the limb are abnormal. Anyone can be born with clubfoot but it tends to occur in families and is slightly more common in boys. Most children born with clubfoot have no other problems, but sometimes it occurs in association with other abnormalities or syndromes.

Although the word 'clubfoot' sounds like something out of a horror movie, the actual appearance is that of a normal foot turned down and inwards. Without treatment, the child would walk on the outer edge of the foot. It is stiff and cannot be brought into normal position.

Clubfoot does not improve with time. It lasts until treated. The diagnosis is made by physical examination, followed by further evaluation by X-ray. An orthopedic surgeon will treat the foot, often using taping, splints, and casts. The foot is gently stretched closer to the correct position and then placed in a cast to hold it there. This procedure is repeated multiple times to bring the foot into the best position possible.

Surgical correction is often needed; treatment may take months or years.

Flat Head

Babies' skulls are very soft and the bones can be affected by pressure. Babies also have weak neck muscles. It is for this reason that the pressure effect of being in a car seat, and the other many modes of transporting babies, has a direct pressure on these soft bones. If the pressure is evenly distributed, the head turns out to be fairly symmetrical. If however the head is not actively placed in different positions there is a tendency to develop a flat spot on one side of the head. This is called positional plagiocephaly or flat head.

A little bit of flattening tends to go away, but more serious flattening may be permanent. It does not affect a baby's brain or development. An easy way of preventing this problem is to change head position routinely. For example, alternate the head of your baby. One day place him with his head at the head of the crib and the next day at the foot of the crib. Make sure the visual stimuli in your baby's room are away from the wall so that he will tend to look into the room and not towards the wall. Tummy time also strengthens the neck and is a useful way to avoid this problem.

With torticollis, the neck muscle is shortened on the one side. This can result from the same causes as flat head syndrome, and the two are often seen together. However, torticollis may develop due to other underlying causes that will require further assessment. Another preventative tool is a neck support that fits around the neck while the baby is in his car seat and this reduces skull pressure.

Immunization

In Canada and North America there is a protocol for immunization against hepatitis B, pneumococcus and Penta with shots given at 2, 4, and 6 months of age. Penta, which means five, protects against Haemophilus influenza, whooping cough, tetanus, diphtheria and polio. In the past there have been some issues and concerns about the link of these shots to diseases such as autism. This is no longer believed to be the case and certainly would not be a reason for me to avoid immunization of my children. I believe that all the shots available in Canada are essential.

Attenuated live viruses such as measles, mumps, rubella and chickenpox (varicella), should all be given at one year of age. We are now also giving a meningitis Menjugate® shot at 2 months and at one year, which gives lifelong immunity. Booster shots for measles, mumps, rubella, Penta and pneumococcus are given at 18 months. Finally a kindergarten booster called Quad (it is the Penta shot minus the Haemophilus influenza) is given at age 4 to 6 yrs.

The most immediate effect of immunization is a localized swelling in the area of injection that is treated with direct cold compresses. In the case of the varicella shot, one can occasionally see some local vesicle or blister appearance that resembles a localized outbreak of chickenpox. We may also see a delayed generalized rash that is due to measles, rubella or chickenpox shots, or a combination. A fever may follow any of these shots and can be treated with Tylenol/acetaminophen.

A fair bit of controversy has existed over the supposed harmful effects of immunization on infants. There was some belief that the preservation of some of the live attenuated viruses in a mercury-derived product called thimerosal was linked to autism. This has never been proven, but to remove this concern all the live attenuated vaccines in Canada are now free of this agent. Whooping cough vaccine may result in a significant fever resulting in a febrile seizure. This has also been modified, so that the risk has now been removed.

Consequently, my recommendation is immunize your kids. This is why Canada has one of the lowest morbidity/mortality rates in the world—because of the excellent free immunization program available for all Canadians.

One last note on immunization that comes at a very exciting time is the introduction of a new immunization program into Canada and the USA in 2006. This is Merck's oral rotavirus vaccine. Rotavirus is one of the leading causes of dehydration and death due to vomiting diarrhea and high fever. It occurs in all parts of the world, and occurs in ages 6-35 months regardless of nutrition, effective hand washing and hygiene. This new vaccine is safe and effective. The most convenient way of fitting this oral vaccine into the current schedule is to administer it along with the 2, 4, and 6 month routine immunization. Discuss this with your doctor at the one month visit.

Crying Baby

Your baby is crying. Why? And what can you do? The checklist says to ask what type of cry it is? As you learn more about your baby, you will recognize the different cries. I know that this sounds crazy, but there are *urgent* cries and *non-urgent* cries. Urgent is usually a cry of severity—I need you now, I am in pain or I am very upset about something. The non-urgent cries are of fussiness—I am hungry, I am thirsty, I have a dirty diaper, I have gas, I need comforting.

At the beginning, it is sometimes confusing for everyone, because for your baby, *everything* is a big deal. Let's face it; the kid has floated around in this warm bath. Life has been good. It has been dark and relaxing, with no stress, and no work needed. Just lying back and being fed directly through a tube attached to the abdomen. This lifeline has provided food and oxygen with no effort required, so your baby has been taking it very easy. Now she's born, everything is a huge deal. The fluid is gone, so now there is this feeling of touch, which really can be quite obtrusive. Then there are all the loud noises and bright lights. Worst of all, there is this work thing called breathing and feeding which require an awful lot of effort.

These new things and feelings from within—gas—and from without—touch, pain, sensation—can all cause distress in your baby. She communicates this by crying. So learn your baby well, and remember that most often crying is more about the new things she is experiencing than about really needing something.

Breathing Patterns

You are sitting and gazing over at your awesome, lightly covered newborn. Hang on! She's not breathing. A sick nauseating panic overcomes you. You race to pick up the phone to dial 911, or…. (You must be thinking as you're reading this that I'm sick! I should not be writing such a tale of woe. Relax. The story gets better.) Meanwhile, you gaze back at your baby, and you notice she's started to breathe in a very shallow and slow irregular way. You heave a sigh of relief. Then the breathing becomes faster and deeper, and did I mention faster and then—it stops. Panic? Or … not? Wait—now she's not breathing again!

Guess what. In a few seconds the whole cycle will start again. This type of breathing is called Cheyne-Stokes breathing and if you do a Google search you will see that this type of breathing is pretty serious in adults. In newborns, not only is it common, it is expected. But it still is a concern for many parents and is often the occasion of a special doctor visit.

Babies breathe like this because part of the brain is still immature, and during sleep it resumes a primitive pattern. As the baby matures, so does the brain and this type of primitive sleep induced breathing will disappear.

Sleeping Positions

Sudden Infant Death Syndrome (SIDS) is thought to occur when infants are placed in soft bedding, where there is a pillow or fluffy toy, and the infant asphyxiates due to lack of oxygen. This is more likely in a baby who lies on their stomach, and according to the latest research, placing your baby on his back reduces the risk for SIDS. Parents often raise concerns that they are unable to keep their baby on his back. I figure if he's that mobile, he's unlikely to run into a problem with oxygen supply. My concern is always that if a newborn who is lying on his back regurgitates, he might breathe in milk and choke. I actually prefer rolling a towel on each side of the baby and wedging him so that he sleeps sideways between the towels without rolling.

Sleeping Pattern

Do not confuse sleeping pattern with sleeping position. This means your baby's sleeping routine. Initially babies dictate their routine—they have relatively short waking periods, during which they feed, and then they sleep. The ideal is that they feed every 2 hours during the day and every 3 hours at night. This will usually result in a healthy weight gain of 4 to 7 ounces average per week. Babies who gain more than this while breast- or bottle-feeding are never a concern. Babies who tend not to gain should be watched closer for a feeding or medical underlying problem. In some case the problem is not the baby but the parent, for example, not enough milk is produced or provided, or perhaps the schedule is not aggressive enough.

Once the baby matures, a schedule is established. Up until 4 months we can expect a baby to require feeds at night. There will come a time when the baby does not need a night feed, but wakes up more for insecurity than hunger needs. Then you will have to learn to distinguish true hunger from a soothing suckle, and you will have to try and help make this transition a pleasant process.

I can't even begin to estimate how many times a week I see a fatigued parent who is finally at their wit's end and needs advice for their now-older infant or toddler. They recognize that the child is no longer truly hungry, so they try to break the established pattern, which is extremely difficult.

It is often a humbling experience. The child's needs are no longer being met in that the parents are not answering their infant's demands. If this sounds familiar, then you've been there or you're still there. As parents, we've all been there.

So it's the middle of the night and you're faced with a kid screaming blue murder, *and tonight's the night!* Come hell or high water you're going to break the pattern, 'cause you're back at work now, and you need your sleep, and you are tired of tonight being the night *for the last three months!* So, you've read all the psychology books, you've watched Supernanny and NANNY 911 on TV, and you're *ready!*

You say goodnight to your darling, and you are now half way out the room, and you are moving really fast now because you know what is about to happen. Your darling stands up and begins to scream. The neighbors and the rest of the block are about to lynch you, and it is time to stop this.

Ok. Let's roll the clock back to the present. Your 4-monther has not yet started this pattern, so, let's set this straight, today, on the first go-around.

You will make sure that your baby is fed and full and content. Bind her securely in a blanket and lay her down in the crib. Make sure she is not too warm and not too cold. Leave some kind of ambient light on, and ambient soft music, if you wish. If you are thinking of rocking your baby to sleep, *don't. Do not rock her to sleep!.*

I know this sounds awfully cruel and inhumane. I am hoping that you can do this while your baby is awake. The rocking thing is fine, but not to get your baby to go to sleep. This is the first step to creating the dependence of the toddler. It sets up the precedent that the only way this kid is going down is with you rocking her to sleep.

Once you are out of the room, your baby may fuss and cry but you are not to go back unless she is truly distressed.

I hope that this is all you will need to do for now. If she continues to cry for more than 10 minutes or if she goes to sleep and then wakes up in 1 to 2 hours and starts to cry, then you can go into the room. Make sure that she is not crying for any other reason such as a poopy diaper, but do not take her out of the crib unless there is a reason to, like changing the poopy diaper. In a very mellow tone, tell your baby that everything is okay, that you love her, and to go to sleep.

Right from the start we are giving a very clear message. There is no confusion here.

Babies and toddlers are confused if we tell them to go to sleep, they cry, and we then come to their rescue a few minutes later, taking them out of the crib. Their cry elicits a response in us, so they know that if they cry or scream, we will answer their call. The baby is conditioning us: he or she cries and we respond. Once this pattern is set, it is tough to break. My approach is to get it right from the start.

In a situation where you have tried this, and it has failed, it is often because the child is older. They are standing and screaming, or sometimes trying to climb out of the crib.

At this stage you may need to take a seat at the side of the crib. She is probably at a developmental stage where you can explain to her what is about to happen. Be clear that it is sleep time. Tell your child that you love her, and tell her to lie down. Do not stimulate her with mobiles or toys in the crib, although you can leave on some soothing music and ambient light, and then leave. If the display begins, then you need to go back. Do not show that this is upsetting you.

Be firm and again state it is sleep time. Do not remove her from the crib. If she is standing tell her to lie down or lay her down.

If this escalates to the point where the child is climbing out of bed to invade your space, you need to be present in the room to prevent this. If this is to succeed, your role is to not interact at all in any way, either verbal or by eye contact way. Your job is to sit at the crib and to be invisible until she tries to climb out of the crib. Then you correct the situation, by stating again that it is sleep time, time to lie down and go to sleep—oh, and that you love her.

Do not give in.

Dress

When dressing your baby, ask yourself how *you* are going to dress. If it's warm out, you are going to dress lightly; the opposite if it's cold. Now multiply that by two for your baby. If it's cold out, and you're going to wear a jacket, your baby needs far more. And remember that if you are hot they are even hotter. Most babies are usually appropriately dressed for cold, but overdressed for heat.

Car Seat

According to the Insurance Corporation of British Columbia, which echoes many motor vehicle insurance companies in North America, infant seats are used in a rear-facing position from birth to one year of age. These seats face backwards in the back seat and are attached with an adult seat belt using a locking clip. This type of seat is used for infants weighing up to 9 to 10 kg (20 to 22 lb).

If the baby is heavier, then you should upgrade to a convertible seat that is placed in the rear-facing position. Convertible seats are good for weights up to16 kg (35 lb). Many child seats indicate they can be used forward facing when the child is between 9 to 10 kg. However, it is much safer to keep your child in a rear-facing seat until she is at least one year of age.

When your child is between the ages of 1 and 4 1/2 years old, and weighs between 20 lb and 40 lb, you can put her in a forward-facing convertible seat with a tether. Combination harness-booster seats are available for taller children up to 48 pounds and between 1 and 4 1/2 years. Booster seats are used for children aged 4 1/2 to 8 years.

Always remember to place an infant/child in a seat that is not close to an airbag to avoid potential injuries arising from the force of activation of the airbag.

Travel

Babies tend to be excellent little travelers. The eternal question once a baby is born is, "How soon can we travel or fly?" The answer is—any time. Babies love motion so car travel is very easy. Air travel is just as easy. It becomes more challenging when they are toddlers. The only challenge for infants is the ascent and the descent. Both of these will cause pressure changes within the aircraft, resulting in pressure behind the eardrum. A good way of overcoming this is to let them cry. This fixes the pressure problem. A more civil way is to let them drink from breast, bottle or cup, depending on age, or to chew gum.

Standing

I am frequently asked if it is okay to allow a baby to stand with support, for fear that it may cause the bones to bend. Fortunately babies have calcified bones that make them solid and therefore as soon as a baby is capable of standing, my advice is to go for it. Babies usually like standing, and often enjoy jumping as young as 6 to 8 weeks if correctly supported in a harness. The neck also needs to have a reasonable tone. If it does not, it should have some support.

Exercise

Babies can exercise at a very early stage as they have been mobile and floating in a body of water for 38 weeks. Thus water-baby exercise programs are encouraged. Babies should be given a daily tummy-time program where they are placed on their stomachs over an increasing period of time so that they can improve their back muscle tone. This enables them to get used to lying in a position other than on the back and will usually result in a better likelihood of becoming a crawler. Babies who are not placed on their stomachs and come to dislike this position usually do not become crawlers.

Bedwetting and Urinary Problems

Nocturnal enuresis or bedwetting may be seen in children over the age of 6 and up until age 12 (and then sometimes beyond). Often parents are concerned that their 3 or 4 year old is wetting the bed. Remember that kids who are newly toilet-trained still have difficulty with their central control. There is nothing wrong with them. This is why they may still have accidents during the day, and certainly at night.

My initial approach is to make sure that there is no underlying pathology. This is usually indicated in toddlers who have been dry and accident-free for many months and are suddenly wet all the time. A urinary sample should be analyzed for pus and blood and then sent for culture and sensitivity. If the sample shows signs of infection, this should be treated, and the child should be assessed for underlying causes such as congenital renal or bladder problems. Other systemic disease such as diabetes should be excluded.

A common cause of frequent urination without an obvious cause is due to what I call high-soap concentration baths. Perhaps your 3-year-old has a bubble bath she enjoys every night with a fish-shaped bar of soap she chases for 30 minutes in the tub. This high concentration of soap can cause a chemical irritation to the urethra (urethritis) resulting in an acute onset of burning with urination and frequent urination (called frequency). The treatment is simple—turf all the bubbles and soap. Do not wash the perineal area (including the penis or vagina) with soap. It's unnecessary. Just a simple wash with cloth and water is all that is needed for perineal care.

If your child is only having problems at night, some of the measures that you can try initially are to restrict fluids in the evening, especially 2 to 3 hours prior to bed. Also, pee your child before you turn in for the night. If, in spite of this, consistent urinary incontinence continues, further tests may be warranted.

Making Strange

A baby makes strange when she suddenly notices that the person she is looking at is not familiar to her. She gets that look on her face and starts to cry. The look we are talking about is the vacant look with a frown. Her eyes then dart back towards the familiar face and she often pouts before she cries. She will sometimes try to get away, even though she is too young to physically take off.

Parents are often concerned about this behaviour, but making strange is actually a good thing. First it shows that your baby recognizes a stranger even if it's Grandpa. It also reassures us that the baby is bonded with his parents. If at 9 months a baby is happy to climb into my arms and has no second thoughts about allowing me to carry him out of the examining room, then I have concerns that he has an attachment disorder. This is something that we recognize in infants from orphanages. As a result of neglect, they detach emotionally and have great difficulty attaching to a parent.

Temper Tantrums

A normal aspect of child development is about to surface—temper tantrums. They begin when your child is about 1 year old, worsen at 2 and are completed, we hope, by the time your child is 3 years old. Older children will use this behaviour if it has worked for them in the past.

Temper tantrums are the result of frustration. They occur if a child is unable to get something. This often starts out innocently with a toddler resisting something that she either does not understand, or understands but is unable to express. They also occur in toddlers who are testing out their independence only to find out that there are constraints to what they can and cannot do.

Some tactics may be used to avoid tantrums, and these may include:

♦ Reward your child with attention for positive behaviour.
♦ Give her some control over little things by giving choices.
♦ Make those off-limit objects disappear: out of sight, out of mind.
♦ Set the stage for success when your child is playing or mastering a new task.
♦ Choose your battles and accommodate when you can but within reason.
♦ Know your child's limits.
♦ Communicate.

In the heat of a tantrum, here are some good tactics:

♦ Keep cool. If you lose your cool, the tantrum often escalates.
♦ If you show frustration, you'll only complicate the problem. Kids know if you are frustrated.

♦ Physical tactics send a message that force and physical punishment is okay. Instead, have enough self-control for both of you.
♦ Lead by example.
♦ Try to understand your child's side.
♦ Use distraction as a technique.
After the tantrum:
♦ Sometimes a child needs to have help or guidance to settle down in the midst of the tantrum.
♦ Never reward a child after a tantrum by giving in. Rather praise her for regaining control.
♦ This is the time to let her know that you love her no matter what.
You need to take the problem to a health professional under the following circumstances:
♦ When the tantrums are getting worse, not better.
♦ If the child is a threat to herself or to those around her.
♦ If the tantrum is evoking feelings from caregivers that result in a negative physical or mental impact on the child.

If your child is in danger of hurting herself or others during a tantrum, remove her to a quiet, safe, place to calm down. This also applies to tantrums in public places.

Milestones

Your baby has so many things to learn; these occur in the form of physical and mental/psychological development. We always gauge babies according to their expected milestones; often we compare our child to others. Sometimes the comparisons do not tell us much and other times they can indicate that there is a motor or learning problem. Always make a note of these concerns for your doctor so that this issue can be dealt with.

Often, the apparent problem is not in fact a problem, because each baby has a definite development timeline that he follows, and this is not always according to the book. Remember too that premature babies are often delayed in their milestones. Some things that your baby should be doing are the following:

At 1 month, he focuses/gazes, he startles to loud or sudden noises, he has established a good suck;

At 2 months, he follows movement with his eyes, he has a variety of sounds and cries, he holds his head up when held at an adult's shoulder, he enjoys being touched and cuddled;

At 4 months, he turns his head toward sounds, he laughs/squeals at his parents, his head is steady, he grasps/reaches;

At 6 months, he follows a moving object, he responds to his own name, he babbles, he rolls from his back to his stomach, or from stomach to back, he sits with support, he brings hands and toys to his mouth;

At 9 months, he looks for hidden toys, he babbles different sounds and to get attention, he sits without support, he opposes thumb and index finger, he reaches to be picked up and held;

At 12 to 13 months, he understands simple requests, e.g., find your shoes, he chatters using 3 different sounds, he crawls or bum shuffles, he pulls to stand/walks holding on, he shows many emotions;

At 18 months, he points to pictures (e.g., show me the cow) and to 3 different body parts, he says at least five words, he picks up and eats finger foods, he walks alone, he stacks at least 3 blocks, he shows affection, he points to show his parents something, he looks at you when talking/playing together;

At 2 years, he has at least 1 new word a week, he uses 2-word sentences, he tries to run, he puts objects into small containers, he copies adults' actions, he continues to develop new skills.

Mom Stuff

Most women experience some problems after delivery with discomfort experienced in the area of the perineum—due to the trauma of pushing out a baby—and in the vicinity—due to hemorrhoids.

Perineal care is important. Spray the area with a spray bottle after urinating or after each bowel movement. This keeps the area clean and therefore reduces any chance of infection. It also minimizes trauma to this sensitive area from wiping with toilet paper.

Exercises

A vaginal delivery causes significant stretching to the vagina and trauma to the surrounding organ structures, namely the ano-rectal area as well as the bladder. This stretching has weakened both the front and back walls of the vagina, which often results in a bladder control problem as a result of the weakness in the front wall. Following vaginal delivery, a cough or sneeze may cause involuntary urination. This is called stress incontinence, and usually improves after several weeks, but you can correct it with Kegel exercises, starting as early as the second day after delivery.

Kegel exercises strengthen the perineal muscles forming the base of the pelvic floor. These muscles, which are weak after delivery, support the bladder, uterus, and bowels.

Lie on your back with your legs relaxed and slightly apart. Contract, or tighten, your pelvic floor muscles by pulling up inside as you would to stop your urine flow. You will feel a slight lifting of the pelvic floor, and it may feel numb in the first several days following birth.

Hold for between 3 to 5 seconds and then relax. Repeat the exercise ten times and try doing ten sessions per day. You can do this in any position while you are doing any other activities. To test these muscles and their strength, try to stop midstream when you are urinating.

The **pelvic tilt** is good for improving back tone and posture. It can also be started two days after delivery.

Lie on your back with your knees bent. Place one hand on your abdomen and one hand under the small of your back. Breathe out as you tighten your abdominal muscles and press the small of your back down towards the bed or exercise mat. You should feel pressure on the hand under the back. Hold this position and breathe normally for a few breaths, and then relax. You may then progress to doing this exercise while sitting and then standing.

A **postural correction** exercise, which can also be started 2 days post-delivery, reintroduces proper posture to your body.

Stand with your back against a wall and your feet about 6 inches away from the base of the wall. Try to stand as tall as possible, tucking your chin in and holding your shoulders slightly back. Tighten your abdominal muscles and do a pelvic tilt, pressing your lower back towards the wall. Your knees should be relaxed and not locked or hyper extended. Then, step away from the wall and practice this position.

At one to two weeks after delivery, you can start the following exercises.

Leg sliding will strengthen your lower abdominal muscles.

Lie on your back with your knees bent. Do a pelvic tilt and maintain the position as you slide one foot along the floor, straightening your knee. Stop sliding your foot when you can no longer hold the pelvic tilt. Then slide your leg back to the starting position and repeat this with the other leg. Once this can be done while keeping a pelvic tilt you are ready to slide both legs at the same time. Return your legs to the starting position one at a time.

Head lifts strengthen your upper abdominal muscles.

Lie on your back with your knees bent. Do a pelvic tilt while at the same time slowly lifting your head off the floor. Breathe out as your abdominals contract. A bulge in the middle of your abdomen, extending from the breastbone to the pelvis, reflects the weakness of the centre part of your abdomen. This is okay—the bulge will become less obvious as the muscles strengthen. One way of reducing this is by crossing your hands over your waist while doing this and pulling towards the midline as you raise your head.

The last two sets of exercises are for stronger abdomens and are done when the first ones have become easier for you. Depending on your fitness level before falling pregnant, you may start them sooner.

Curl ups work the rectus abdominal muscles.

Lie on your back with knees bent. Tuck your chin in and do a pelvic tilt. Lift your head and shoulders and reach towards your knees with both hands. Breathe out while curling up. Slowly return to the start position while breathing in.

Diagonal curl ups strengthen the oblique abdominal muscles.

Lie on your back with your knees bent. Tuck your chin in and do a pelvic tilt. Curl up, lifting your shoulders and reach to the outside of your right knee with both hands. Breathe out while curling up. Hold, then slowly return to the start position while breathing in. Then repeat on the left side.

Lacerations and Tears

If a natural tear has occurred, it is stitched at the time of delivery. Most stitches are made in different layers with a continuous stitch. The most common stitch material, Vicryl®, is synthetic and dissolves on its own. Catgut is an older material and also dissolves on its own.

If you have had an episiotomy, the extent of the cut will usually be worse than a natural tear, it will usually be more painful and take longer to heal.

Tears can be classified according to how bad they are. A first-degree tear involves the mucous membrane only while a second-degree tear involves the muscle as well. If a tear extends to involve the anus, it is called a third-degree tear and is serious in that if it is not repaired properly it can result in anal incontinence. This can result in soiling of underwear and may become an embarrassing problem after the delivery.

Stretch Marks

Striae gravidarum or stretch marks occur due to the stretching of abdominal skin during pregnancy. The elastic fibres of the skin rupture and form curved lines that are red or pink initially; after delivery they become silvery-white.

Only one third of pregnant women develop stretch marks, and it is unusual to see these markings in people who have other causes for enlarged abdomens. People with Cushing's syndrome produce excess glucocorticosteroids, and they develop similar stretch marks. Pregnant woman also produce high amounts of this same hormone.

The only way to prevent stretch marks is to try and minimize the trauma to the elastic tissue. Massage with vitamin-E oil or cocoa butter often works; if this fails, Retin-A or laser treatment may be used after the pregnancy.

Hemorrhoids and Anal Fissures

Hemorrhoids are found in all individuals, in the area of the anal muscle or sphincter. The tissue in this area is vascular in nature, similar to veins. Of the two kinds of hemorrhoid tissue, internal hemorrhoids are found above the anal sphincter and are not visible to the naked eye when they become swollen. External hemorrhoids are found below the anal sphincter, and when they swell they are felt on wiping and are also seen as lumps.

This is one of the most painful problems for women following childbirth. Often, the growing baby in the uterus, and the delivery itself, can cause the hemorrhoid tissue to swell. Also, because of the pressure of the large uterus towards the end, there is often an associated pressure on the rectum, causing constipation and the need to push harder with each bowel movement. This causes the swollen tissue to become worse. Finally, the pushing that occurs at the end almost guarantees that hemorrhoid tissue will swell.

If internal hemorrhoids swell, they can bleed, and blood will be visible on wiping after a bowel movement or in the toilet. Internal hemorrhoids never hurt; it is external hemorrhoids that swell and hurt so much.

Finally, if the stool is hard, it can cause a tear in the anal muscle called a fissure. Often all three problems will occur together.

The treatment for all three problems is the same:

- Eat lots of fibre daily—the best form is in All-Bran® Buds
- Avoid long toilet visits with reading material—*unless, of course, you are reading this book*
- Do not strain
- Wipe using baby wipes—don't waste your money on Tucks® at $8.00 for wafer-size baby wipes that last one bowel movement.

There are many topical products for relief of the pain and they all work. The prescribed hemorrhoid topicals usually have corticosteroids to shrink the inflamed tissue. Some may have an additional anesthetic, which is especially soothing if you have fissures.

The applicators that come with these creams always puzzle me. Most patients have a very sensitive bottom, and now they are expected to insert this big nozzle into an already painful area and to cause even more pain!

I recommend a product called Proctofoam® HC. It's foamy, non-greasy, and easy to apply. It even has an applicator that is of a much more reasonable size when considering options for anal insertion.

Breast Engorgement (or Lack Thereof)

As you begin to breast-feed, you are stimulating the nipples to send a message to the pituitary gland to release prolactin, the hormone that stimulates breast tissue to produce milk. The more the breast is stimulated with feeding the more milk is produced. But sometimes, in spite of all efforts to breast feed, milk just does not come in. If this happens, it's worth renting an electrical pump as a excellent stimulant until the milk comes in. Another alternative is to take Motilium®, or domperidone maleate (not the drink), which is a gastrointestinal drug used to improve sluggish contractions of the bowels. This drug is safe for breastfed babies and causes no side effects but will cause breast milk production.

If your situation is the opposite and you are engorged with too much breast milk, ***do not attempt to pump,*** as this will stimulate even more milk production. You can reduce the engorgement by expressing milk in the shower, or by ensuring sure that your baby is feeding well and with not too long a period between feeds.

If you are not planning to breast feed, the best management is to bind your breasts with a tensor bandage. Do not to stimulate them with any breastfeeding or pumping. The drug Parlodel® is available to turn off the release of prolactin and works well, although it has fallen out of use as it has a small incidence (~0.01%) of stroke, which is naturally a negative incentive.

Mastitis

Mastitis is one of the most common infections seen in breastfeeding mothers and is due to stasis of milk within the breast milk ducts. It is characterized by redness and pain on the involved side. Generalized fever and chills usually warrant a more aggressive approach. Treat it with oral antibiotics such as Keflex®, Ceftin®, or Zithromax®, which are all safe while breastfeeding. Do not stop feeding off that breast, and do not worry that the milk from that side is harmful to your baby.

Prolactin

Prolactin is an interesting hormone because as important as it is in the production of breast milk, it also creates a few additional issues. It is directly responsible for alopecia, which is almost inevitable if you are a breastfeeding mother. The hair loss reverses as soon as you stop breastfeeding.

It also causes sweating, which is another common complaint for breastfeeding mothers. Often lactating mothers complain that they used to smell quite nice, but since they have been breastfeeding, they've noticed a change in body odour. Again, it's due to prolactin.

Finally, often husbands ask if there is a specific reason for his wife or partner to be so loopy. Again, the culprit is prolactin. But on the positive side, think of those 500 calories you burn each day that you are breastfeeding.

While breastfeeding, your periods may be disrupted. You may not have a period at all or you may have a regular period, or you may spot on and off or throughout the cycle. All are considered quite typical while breastfeeding.

Leg Swelling

In the first week following delivery, women often complain that their previously pregnancy-induced swollen ankles (cankles) are now even more swollen. This is the result of the combination of labour, pushing, redistribution of hormones, as well as retention of fluids following the birth. As a rule, ankle swelling resolves within the second week. You should also avoid salt and this should help.

Post-Partum Depression

Post-partum depression is now widely acknowledged; it can occur for up to one year after delivery. It is often due to a predisposition to depression either because of a previous history or a family history. It is, however, seen without any other cause other than having had a baby. It is believed to be partly hormone-induced, but is also due to childbirth itself.

After all, the past 10 months have been filled with excitement at the prospects of this wonderful new bundle of joy, only to find out that the bundle is sometimes no joy at all. It is a commitment, a lifelong change requiring a 24-hour obligation without pay or reward.

So gloom sets in, and there is no fun in this new life with this little parasitical being who continuously needs food, makes noises, poops, pees, and causes sleep deprivation, which only serves to make you more sad and depressed.

The good news is that this condition is treatable by counseling to give you a positive view on this exciting time in your life. You can also take antidepressant drugs that will work within about two weeks of starting them.

Sex

If you had a C- section, with no attempts to have a vaginal birth, then it is unlikely that you have any vaginal trauma. In this case, you may have intercourse once your C-section scar has healed. Just avoid lifting your partner during intercourse.

If you had a vaginal delivery, you will be experiencing some degree of vaginal trauma, whether you needed stitches or not. The time required to heal will depend on a number of factors such as the size of your baby, number of deliveries and how easy this delivery was for you. Consider all these factors before resuming intercourse.

My advice is, don't rush it and tell your partner to go slow and gently. This way you can gauge for yourself whether there is any discomfort or not.

By the sixth week, most patients have healed, although some will have pain with intercourse for as long as up to six months after delivery.

Remember as well, that unless you are planning to fall pregnant again, you will need some form of protection against falling pregnant.

Birth Control

One terrible misconception is that if you breast feed you will not fall pregnant. *This is absolutely untrue.* You can and will fall pregnant, so ask your doctor about the two options available to you. Both are safe while breastfeeding.

The *minipill* is a progesterone-only pill that can be started three weeks prior to having sex and is taken every day without a break. It is still not 100% protective, but when taken in conjunction with breastfeeding, it provides protection that is considered to be almost as good as the combination estrogen/progesterone pill. It can result in three different scenarios when it comes to a period. Because you start it without having first had a period and because you take it daily without a break, you could get your period once a month, or you may not get a period at all, or you may get a period on and off.

Depo-Provera is an injectable progesterone only hormone that is injected into the muscle every 12 to 13 weeks. It will cause your periods to completely disappear by the third shot.

Depo-Provera has three negative aspects. First, you are almost guaranteed to gain weight on the shots; second, Depo-Provera is so effective that when you decide to fall pregnant again, it may take you as long as two years. Third, and very topical, is the pos-

sibility of osteoporosis (thin bones) in association with this drug.
Take all three points into consideration before deciding to take
this method of birth control.

A Final Word

I hope that this book has given you a good summary of what you may expect in the months ahead. My goal has been to provide all newly pregnant women with everything essential to your pregnancy, delivery and initial nurturing of your newborn. I hope to have simplified things for you in one book.

I don't think my work is done. I have enjoyed this opportunity so much that I expect to continue in the future either by expanding on some of the more complex subjects or perhaps with further overviews. I look forward to feedback from everyone reading this book. Please feel free to e-mail me at ableman2223@telus.net.

And finally, I'd like to thank Clélie Rich for her editorial feedback and guidance.

Internet Addresses

For those of you with access to the Internet, here are some helpful websites.

Canadian Institute of Child Health:
www.cich.ca

BabyCenter (a pregnancy and baby site):
www.babycenter.com

Canadian Paediatric Society:
www.cps.ca

Canadian AIDS Society (for HIV/AIDS in pregnancy):
www.cdnaids.ca

Circle of Pregnancy
www.circleofpregnancy.com

La Leche League International:
www.lalecheleague.org

Lamaze International:
www.lamaze.org

MotherRisk (for resources and information on pregnancy):
www.motherisk.com

Health Canada (nutrition and breastfeeding):
www.hc-sc.gc.ca/fn-an/nutrition/child-enfant/infant-nourisson/index_e.html

The Canadian Federation for Sexual Health (Planned Parenthood Federation of Canada):
www.ppfc.ca

Society of Obstetricians and Gynaecologists of Canada:
www.sogc.org

Twins Magazine (Twins and multiple births):
www.twinsmagazine.com

BC Women's Hospital & Health Centre:
www.bcwomens.ca

Index

A

abdominal cavity 26, 27
   muscles 30, 68, 149, 150, 151
Abruptio placentae 33, 79, 80
acupuncture 95
acne 31, 60, 123
AIDS 16, 37, 38
alcohol 14, 16, 25, 26, 32, 55, 84, 111, 122
alopecia 154
amniocentesis 38, 40, 41, 42, 67
amniotic fluid 24, 46, 54, 56, 63, 65, 68, 69, 70, 73, 75, 77, 78, 88, 92, 129
anal fissure 152
   incontinence 151
analgesics
   Demerol® 95, 96
   Entanox® 95
   epidural 96, 97
      bupivicaine and, 96
      fentanyl and, 96
      ropivacaine and, 96
      walking and, 96
   fentanyl 95
   laughing gas 95
   narcotics 95
   nitrous oxide 95
anemia 21, 38, 46, 54, 107
antacids 60
antibiotic ointment 109
antibodies
   in colostrum 112
   blood rhesus 56
antifungal
   oral 128
   vaginal 61, 121

Apgar score 108, 109
arachidonic acid(ARA) 114
attachment disorder 145
augmentation of labour 88, 100
autism 135, 136

B

B vitamins 14
bacon nitrites 22
babies
   acne and, 123
   alcohol and, 26
   bowel movements 39, 118, 125
   breasts of 122
   breathing 138
   breech 44, 133, 134
   care of 109, 110, 111, 115, 118
   clothing of 142
   constipation in 118
   crying 125
   dehydration 119, 120, 121, 137
   development
      full term 147
      embryonic 44
      fetal 44
      second trimester 45
      third trimester 45
   diarrhea 119
   eyes 129
   feeding 111, 114, 115, 118
   fever 131, 132
   overdue 89
   premature 74, 77, 110
   seizures 132
   sex determination 12, 38, 67, 68, 111
   size 69
   skin 123
   temperature 110, 131, 132
   teeth 124
   vomiting 119

F

False labour 83
family history 37, 118, 155
family physician 35
fast foods 24
fennel tea 126
fetal alcohol syndrome (FAS) 25, 26
fetal 25, 38, 43, 44, 45, 46, 50, 55, 56,
    58, 64, 65, 67, 68, 70, 75, 84, 85,
    88, 89, 92, 99, 102, 103
    development 19, 44, 45, 46
    heart rate 67, 68, 75, 84, 92, 103
    monitoring 75, 84, 88, 92, 102, 103
        external 84, 88, 92, 102, 103
        internal 103
    movement 64, 65
        count 65
    viability 38
fibre 61, 153
first prenatal visit 19, 37, 43
first trimester 31, 32, 53, 55
flat head 135
flu shots 64
fluid retention 24, 49
fluoride 117, 118, 124
fluorosis 117, 118, 124
folate 14, 21
fontanelle 130
    anterior 130
    posterior 130
forceps 99, 101, 102, 103
formula feeding 114
foreskin 121, 122
frenulum 115
fruit juice 22
fungal infection 61, 121, 128
    oral 128
    vaginal 61, 121

G

galactosemia 109
genital herpes 47
gestational diabetes 24, 43, 47, 48, 54
getting up 27
glucose tolerance test (GTT) 48
gripe water 126
Group B strep (GBS) 46, 89
growth and development 38, 43, 44, 46

H

hair 44, 60, 68, 98, 123, 154
    growth 60
    loss 154
headaches 27, 50
head circumference 92
health care provider 69
heart failure 48, 50
heartburn 50, 60
hemoglobin 46, 47, 54
hemorrhage 48, 56, 79, 80, 81, 100, 104
    labour and, 80, 81
    post delivery 100, 104
hemorrhoids 61, 148, 152
    external 152
    internal 152
hepatitis 16, 37, 38, 135
herpes 47
hiccups 64
HIV 16, 37, 38
home pregnancy test 19
hormones 58, 60, 62, 63, 155
    effects on baby 44, 114, 122
    effects on mother 60, 62, 63
hot tub 93
human chorionic gonadotrophin (hCG)
20, 23, 39, 55
hyperemesis gravidarum 23
hypertension 37, 44, 48, 49, 80
hypnosis 95

hypoxia 49

I

immature lungs 45, 74, 110
immunization 64, 136
immunoglobulins 112
   passive 112
implantation 38, 54, 79
incompetent cervix 56, 77
infections 56, 61, 128, 129, 131, 154
   amniotic fluid 56, 63, 65, 77
   breast 154
   urinary 77, 144
   uterus 46, 56, 63
insulin 48
internal fetal monitoring 103
introitus 98
intrauterine device (IUD) 16
intrauterine growth retardation (IUGR) 54
iron 14, 21, 46, 54, 114
iron supplement 114

J

jaundice 110, 126, 127, 128
   breast milk 127
   Kramer' classification of, 128
   pathology and 127
   phototherapy and, 127, 128
   physiology and, 126, 127
   treatment of 127, 128

K

Kegel exercise 29, 149
kidney stone 93, 94

L

labour 12, 25, 26, 29, 30, 32, 36, 46, 47,
   56, 64, 65, 69, 70, 71, 73, 74, 75,
   77, 78, 79, 80, 83, 84, 85, 87, 88,
   89, 90, 91, 92, 93, 94, 95, 96, 97,
   100, 101, 102, 103, 104, 105, 112,
   130, 155
   augmentation 88, 100
   impending 70, 71, 90
   induction 65, 89
   preterm 25, 56, 73, 74
   premature 77
   Stage, 1st 90
   Stage, 2nd 90, 91, 97, 98, 99,
      100, 101
   Stage, 3rd 90, 104, 105
laceration 151
lanolin 113
lanugo 44
large baby 24
last menstrual period (LMP) 20
latching on 115
laying down
leg cramps 31, 59
leg swelling 62, 63, 155
   after delivery 63, 155
   pregnancy and, 62
leucorrhoea 62
ligament 57, 58, 68
liver function tests 49, 50
lovemaking 63
low birth weight 25, 110, 111

M

magnesium sulphate 50
making strange 145
mask of pregnancy 60
mastitis 154
massage 58, 94, 129, 152
maternity vitamins 25, 46
meconium 88
medical history 16, 37, 42
measles 16, 64, 136

meat 12, 14, 15, 16, 22, 118
medication 13, 23, 31, 32, 48, 73, 94
   Accutane® 31
   ace inhibitor (antihypertensive) 31
   anticoagulation
      Coumadin® 31
   anticonvulsant
      dilantin 31
      phenytoin 31
      Valproic acid 31
   antihistamines
      ephedrine 32
      pseudoephedrine 32
   birth control 157
   contraindicated 13, 31, 33
   Diclectin® 23
   during labour 73, 95-96
   for nausea & vomiting 23
   ibuprofen 32, 132
   Labetalol 48
   lithium 31
   Losec® 31
   methyl-dopa 48
   pain relief 93, 94, 95, 96, 97, 104
   Paxil®, 32
   pregnancy and, 31, 32
   Quinine 31
   SSRI 31, 32
   Zantac® 32
Medium Chain Acyl-coA Dehydrogenase deficiency (MCAD) 109
membrane rupture 46, 48, 56, 73, 75, 77,
      78, 88
   stripping 65
mental retardation 109
mercury 22, 136
   seafood 22
milk lactation 111, 112
   formula 114, 115, 116, 117, 119, 127,
      128
   production 111, 112

   unpasteurized 16
midwives 36, 68
milestones 147
minipill 157
miscarriage 19, 22, 32, 33 37, 41, 42,
      55, 56
Mogen circumcision 121
morning sickness 23, 31
Motilium® (domperidone) 117, 154
mucous membranes 130
mucous plug 71
multiple births 111

N

narcotics 95
nasal stuffiness/congestion 59, 129
natural childbirth 71 87, 90, 92
nausea 21, 23, 27, 46, 53
neural tube defects 21, 39, 40
Neutrogena soap 123
nonstress test (NST) 49
nipples 111, 113, 119, 122, 153
nitrites 22
nocturnal enuresis 144
nuchal thickness 43
nursing
   formula 113, 114
   natural 111
nutrition
   fetal 112
   maternal 14

O

obstetricians 35, 53
obstructed labour 101
occipito-posterior position (OP) 98
older mothers
ophthalmic infection 129
omega fatty acids
   omega 3 114

ring of fire 98
Rotavirus 120, 137
rubella 16, 38, 64, 136

S

sacroiliac joint 58
saline nose drops 130
salt retention 54, 62
sausage nitrites 22
schedule 23, 35, 112, 113, 139
seafood 22
sex 38, 44, 46, 63, 67, 68, 84, 93, 111,
    122, 156, 157
seborrheic dermatitis 123
second trimester 53
seizure 48, 136
Sudden Infant Death Syndrome
(SIDS) 125, 139
show 71
skin
    baby 45, 115, 120, 121, 123, 124, 126,
        127
    mother 60
sleep pattern 139-142
smoking 14, 16, 25, 73
snore 59
solid foods in babies 118
soother 125
spina bifida 21, 39, 41
spontaneous rupture of membranes
(SROM) 75, 88
sports 26, 119
stretch marks 152,
sterilize 113
stitches 151, 156
sugar 43, 47, 62, 119
surgery 134
    Caesarian section 47, 50, 69, 80, 81,
               89, 93, 101, 102,
               103, 104, 156

D & C 104
retained products 104, 105
termination 40
stool 114, 119, 120, 153
strabismus 129
striae gravidarum 151
supplementation with
    potassium 59
    calcium 59
    magnesium 59
surfactant 74
suture 130
syphilis 16, 38
sweating 155
swollen ankles 27, 155

T

tantrums 146, 147
Tay-Sachs disease 37
tea
    herbal 33, 126
    regular 33
tear ducts
    massage and, 129, 130
tear 151
    1st degree 151
    2nd degree 151
    3rd degree 151
termination of pregnancy (TOP) 40
thalassemia 37
third trimester 31
thimerosal 136
thrush 128
thumb sucking
tooth decay 117, 124, 125
tongue-tied 115
Torticollis 113, 135
toxemia 43, 47, 48, 49
toxoplasmosis 16
travel

air 64, 143
car 64, 143
transition 45, 96, 139
transverse lie 46
trimester 24, 31, 32, 53, 54, 55, 58, 64
1st 31, 32, 53, 55
2nd 53
3rd 31
triple screen test 38-43
false positive 38, 41, 42, 43
negative 41
trisomy
trisomy 18 39, 40
trisomy 21 39-43
tuna 22
twin pregnancies 23, 33, 38

U

ultrasound 33, 38, 41, 43, 44, 45, 46, 49,
54, 55, 67, 75, 78, 80, 81, 85,
89, 91, 133
ultraviolet light 127
umbilical cord 47, 85, 104, 107
undercooked meat 22
poultry 22
underweight 23, 24
urethritis (chemical) 144
uric acid crystals 121
urinary crystals 121
urinary
frequency 144
incontinence 145, 149
infection (UTI) 62, 63, 77
urine pregnancy test 20
uterine biometric monitor 84, 88
contractions 74, 75

V

vacuum 101, 103, 126
vaginal birth after caesarian section

(VBAC) 103, 104
vaginal discharge 61, 62, 71, 74
vaginal herpes 47
valium 49
varicose veins 63
VDRL test 38
vernix caseosa 45
vertex 104
vigamox 129
vitamins
vitamin A 25
vitamin B 14
vitamin D 25, 117
vitamin K 109
vomiting 27, 119, 120, 137

W

walking 27, 39, 96, 126
water breaking 46, 56
weight gain 22, 23, 24, 49, 53, 54, 117,
139
loss 53, 54, 115, 116, 117

X

X-ray pelvimetry 91

Y

yeast infection 61, 128
oral 128
vaginal 61, 121

Z

zinc 14, 120, 121

ISBN 141209481-X

9 781412 094818